The Perricone Prescription

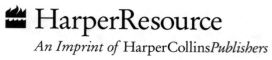

HarperResource

An Imprint of HarperCollins*Publishers*

The Perricone Prescription

A Physician's
28-Day Program
for Total Body and
Face Rejuvenation

Nicholas Perricone, M.D.

FIRST EDITION

Designed by Joy O'Meara

Library of Congress Cataloging-in-Publication Data

Perricone, Nicholas.
  The perricone prescription : a physician's 28-day program for total body and face rejuvenation / Nicholas Perricone.—1st ed.
    p.   cm.
  Includes index.
  ISBN 0-06-018879-0
  1. Beauty, Personal.   2. Face—Care and hygiene.   I. Title.

RA778 .P37 2002
646.7'26—dc21   2002023284

02   03   04   05   06   RRD   10   9

Dedicated to my revered teacher and mentor
at the Henry Ford Medical Center, Detroit, Michigan,
the late Clarence S. Livengood, M.D.
Chairman Emeritus, Department of Dermatology, Henry Ford Hospital
Former Executive Director of the American Board of Dermatology

CONTENTS

Acknowledgments

I would like to extend a warm thank you to the great many friends and colleagues who have generously assisted me, including:

A special thanks to Anne Sellaro, agent, friend, collaborator and executive producer, whose matchless skills, enthusiasm and creativity prove that all things are possible

My friends and colleagues at Yale University School of Medicine for their continued kindness and support of my work

Michigan State University College of Human Medicine

Larry DeNardis, Jacqueline Koral, and Thad Henry of University of New Haven

Department of Dermatology Henry Ford Hospital

Dan Cody

Tony Tiano and everyone at Santa Fe Ventures

Diane Reverand

The HarperCollins team: Jennifer Brehl, Megan Newman, Kate Stark, Shelby Meizlick, Josh Marwell and the entire sales force, Donna Ruvituso, Diane Aronson, and Robin Bilardello

David Vigliano

Neil Mahrer, Sylvia Bennett and the team at Public Broadcasting System (PBS-TV)

Christiane Northrup, MD

Stephen Sinatra, MD, FACN, FACC

Harry Preuss, MD, FACN

My dedicated staff at Clinical Creations—thanks for all your support and hard work

My wonderful children Nicholas, Jeff, and Caitlin

My parents, who made all of this possible

To Madeleine Perricone, for her invaluable research and insight, greatly contributing to my many ongoing research projects

To Vincent Perricone, for support and friendship over the years

INTRODUCTION

We are fortunate to live at a time when science has extended our lives significantly. Advances in research and medical treatment promise us unprecedented longevity. According to the United States Social Security Administration, at present the average life expectancy at birth is 73.9 years for men and 79.6 years for women. MIT recently released a report on laboratory experiments affecting the genes that control aging. According to the *New York Times,* if a drug were ever developed from these studies that worked on humans, we would enjoy a life span of up to 170 years, most of it in perfect health. And, although such longevity is not yet a reality for humans, we can expect to be fully functioning, vibrant, and productive for decades beyond members of our parents' generation.

Cardiologists have learned the mechanics of the heart and circulation, and have developed techniques for the prevention and reversal of heart disease. Neuroscientists and neurologists are breaking new ground in the understanding of the delicate balance of neurotransmitters and hormones in our brains and the deficiencies and excess that cause aging. Oncologists and cancer researchers are making great strides in the fight against cancer. There are countless breakthroughs in the treatment of chronic diseases like diabetes, Parkinson's, arthritis, and more.

Science is making new inroads in conquering disease and keeping our physical systems and organs in good working order longer than ever. But this is all internal progress. Your skin—visible to all—is your largest organ, and when skin ages, it announces its condition to the world. Although we cannot stop the progression of the years, we can stop skin from wrinkling, sagging, and dulling. During my years as an assistant clinical professor of dermatology at Yale University School of Medicine, and my fifteen years in private practice and research, I have cared for thousands of patients in my private practice. My research has led to a variety of treatments that prove that looking and feeling old is now an option. You can reverse and certainly prevent visible skin damage and put your best face forward. Being wrinkle free for life is achievable if you follow the 28-Day Program in this book.

If you are like most readers you have probably already thumbed through the before-and-after photographs in this book. I made the decision to use ordinary people with busy lives to participate in the 28-Day Wrinkle-Free Program. One group of subjects consisted of volunteers from my publisher's New York office. Forty men and women followed the Wrinkle-Free Program for a month. We documented the changes and have included a selection of photographs in these pages.

In addition, Johnson & Johnson conducted clinical trials of DMAE (dimethylaminoethanol) with astonishing statistical and visual results, which I cover in detail in Chapter Five. They, too, took before-and-after photographs of the participants. Now, these are not glamorous shots. In fact, they were taken in a very controlled, clinical setting: that of the photo studio at the Johnson & Johnson headquarters in New Jersey. The camera and the lights are fixed in place, and the chairs in which the subjects sit to be photographed are fastened to the floor. A brace holds each woman's chin. That ensures that her head is in the same position in the before as in the after shot. There are no tricks with lighting or camera angle. Even the women's hair is blocked from the photos. These are not fashion layouts, and the women are not models, but when you see the improvements in their faces you will be dazzled.

Before you begin my full program, you will want to try the Three-Day Nutritional Face-lift. If you eat only what I suggest for just three days, you will see an immediate improvement in your appearance as well as experience a boost in energy. I demonstrated this three-day miracle on *Good Morning America,* and the results caused a sensation. My first book, *The Wrinkle Cure,* became an overnight, runaway bestseller. You can use this three-day diet whenever you want to look and feel your best. Whether you are preparing for a job interview, a special date, a big social event, or a business presentation, the Three-Day Nutritional Face-lift will ensure that you'll be radiant and energetic.

I recommend that you test this three-day diet plan immediately. Once you do, I know its remarkable effects will inspire you to read on to find out why you are looking and feeling so terrific. After all, once you experience firsthand how well the plan works in just three short days, imagine the transformation you can achieve with the 28-Day Program!

In Chapter Two, "The Inflammation-Aging Connection," I will explain the scientific theory behind my work. My research has shown that the signs of aging—including wrinkling, crepey skin, sagging jawline and jowls, drooping eyelids, under-eye bags and puffiness—are all the results of inflammation. Inflammation is a probable culprit, a contributor to most major diseases and degenerative conditions, from cancer to Alzheimer's, arthritis to stroke. Proinflammatory diets, exposure to sunlight, environmental pollutants, and a host of other agents assault our cells and cause them to generate inflammatory chemicals. This subclinical inflammation goes on day after day, year in and year out, leading to numerous disease states as well as the disease of aging. Yes, aging is a disease—a chronic, uniformly progressive, inflammatory disease that is always fatal. In Chapter Two, I explain how inflammation occurs on a cellular level and detail my search for powerful anti-inflammatories—antioxidants that stop inflammation and repair the damage. If you can prevent and stop inflammation, you can prevent and stop the signs of aging.

At this point, you will be ready to learn about the four aspects of the 28-Day Program: diet, supplements, skin care, and exercise. Chapter Three provides a full explanation of the Wrinkle-Free Diet, which is composed of anti-inflammatory foods. It's true: you are what you eat. And what you eat can rob you of your youth. The wrong foods are responsible for rapid, premature aging; a tired, drawn, and doughy complexion; flaccid, weak muscle tone; wrinkled, leathery, dried-out looking facial skin; fatigue; and poor brain power. Whoever invented the Happy Meal was not on the road to the fountain of youth! My diet promotes youthful, wrinkle-free, toned skin and sharp muscle definition. Eating the wrinkle-free way will bring back those high cheekbones, defined jawline, and rosy glow. You will experience increased vitality, sharpened cognitive and problem-solving skills, and improved memory. The Wrinkle-Free Diet will become your new way of life!

In Chapter Four, I review the supplements that will enhance your transformation and outline my comprehensive supplement program. My aim is to rebuild and rejuvenate your body and skin from the inside out.

By using targeted antioxidants, amino acids, vitamins, and minerals, you will accomplish a host of things, from sharpening your brain power to repairing cells, from burning fat to increasing muscle tone, from restoring memory to heightening libido. Good health and beautiful skin go hand in hand, and the correct supplements can help you achieve and maintain both.

Chapter Five deals with skin care to combat aging. I discuss my own research and the discoveries I have made and incorporated into the creation of topical treatments. When anti-inflammatories are applied to the skin, the results are nothing short of miraculous. Working from the outside in, these powerful potions produce striking short-term and cumulative long-term improvements in skin quality. I will explain how vitamin C ester, alpha lipoic acid, DMAE, PPC (polyenylphosphatidyl choline), super vitamin E (tocotrienol), and olive oil polyphenols penetrate, strengthen, and refresh your skin cells. I recommend a broad range of skin care products that are accessible to everyone. You will find specific directions for your own skin type, with special advice for African-American, Mediterranean, Latino, and Asian skin.

It's just not possible to stay radiant without regular exercise. Chapter Six, "Go for the Glow," covers the three elements of fitness: cardiovascular, muscle strength, and flexibility. Exercise of almost any kind has a powerful, positive, and anti-inflammatory effect on all our cells. This chapter presents a simple plan for incorporating exercise into your life. Exercise need not be drudgery, as my complete fitness plan will prove to you.

In Chapter Seven, it all comes together in an easy-to-follow 28-Day plan. Simply follow the program, and you will see and feel extraordinary changes in your body and your outlook. Once you're in the swing of it, you'll feel so great you won't even be tempted to stray, and you'll want to adopt the Perricone Wrinkle-Free Program as a way of life.

I will give you a glimpse of the exciting direction in which research is headed—and some of the amazing advances you can expect to see in the not so distant future in Chapter Eight.

Finally, let's not forget the appendices that include twenty-seven delicious—and simple—recipes that will make eating the wrinkle-free way even more pleasurable; and resources for skin care products, vitamin supplements, and antiaging doctors.

Our society is obsessed by youth. At my lectures, I often ask the women in the audience, "How many of you feel that your husband or boyfriend looks younger than you do? Is he aging better than you are?" Without fail, the majority of women raise their hands. The fact is, most women do not age as well as men. But it's important to remember that the signs of aging do not afflict only women; the Perricone Program is as beneficial to men as it is to women. In fact, in my antiaging practice, my male patients are equal in number to my female patients. The good news is that *The Perricone Prescription* will provide you with a proven program to reverse the many signs of premature aging and stop its progress. The smooth skin that contributes so much to your youthful appearance does not have to be lost during mid-life and beyond. If you follow my 28-Day Wrinkle-Free Program, you will rejuvenate your face and your body, and will see for yourself that aging is an option.

Since I am an active researcher, your feedback is important to me. If you would like to comment on my program and its effect on you, please feel free to e-mail me at www.nvperriconemd.com.

I hope that you are now eager to get started. The Three-Day Nutritional Face-lift that follows will get you on the fast track to restoring ageless, supple, and radiant skin.

—Nicholas Perricone, M.D.
January 2002

1

Dr. Perricone's Three-Day Nutritional Face-lift

Each morning I follow the same routine. Once I get to the office, I drink a large glass of water and don a crisply starched, white lab coat. I sit down at my desk and glance over my schedule for the day, study the latest results of my patients' lab tests, and read the preparatory notes for my first consultation.

And each day I am filled with the same eager anticipation—the challenge of helping my patients turn their lives around. Even though I have been in active practice for more than a decade, the rewards of being a dermatologist never fade, because the results are so visible. Physicians who specialize in internal medicine or cardiology, for example, know that if their treatment recommendations are followed, lives can be prolonged and saved. But they can never experience the thrill of seeing a patient return with beautiful, healthy skin, after suffering—sometimes for years—from a disfiguring condition that destroyed the quality of his or her life. The Three-Day Nutritional Face-lift is a gift—one that will allow you to experience the joy of transformation. If you follow the plan in this chapter, you will see visible results with your own eyes.

The promise of a visible difference in your looks in just three days may seem too good to be true. But if you eat the wrinkle-free way for even a short period of time, you will experience dramatic changes not only in how you look but also in how you feel. You should consider this a test drive. Before you commit to the full month-long program, try the simple three-day plan outlined in this chapter.

The Three-Day Nutritional Face-lift focuses on food, the most powerful ally in the fight against wrinkles, sags, and loss of skin tone. Once you see and feel the results you will realize that there is a face-lift in your fridge. The three-day diet presented in this chapter reflects the fundamental concepts of my research on inflammation and aging. With science supporting my recommendations, I am confident that this three-day plan will work for you as it has for so many of my patients.

Jill, a forty-five-year-old former model who is now an executive at a financial management company, came to me for an antiaging consultation. As I entered the examination room and introduced myself, my first impression was that she looked thin and fragile. Even her beautiful smile could not hide how drawn her face was.

When I asked some general background questions about her overall health, she said that in addition to being worried about looking old before her time, her energy levels had hit rock bottom. Jill explained that she had become lethargic; she was always tired and frequently depressed. Although the depression was not severe, she felt the sparkle had gone out of her life. Jill also reported a major loss in her libido, placing a strain on her relationship with her husband. Concerned, Jill had recently made an appointment with her internal medicine physician, who gave her a clean bill of health after a comprehensive physical examination. She was now consulting me to see if a different approach could alleviate her symptoms. I asked Jill about her diet and was not surprised to find that she was severely limiting her caloric intake and was eating almost no protein. Jill admitted that during her years as a model she ate very little and became bulimic in her efforts to keep her weight down. Although she was no longer modeling, her bulimia persisted. At five feet nine inches tall, Jill currently weighed a scant 110 pounds. In fact, like Jill, many women are nutritionally deprived. As a result of their unique brain chemistry, women tend to eat far less protein than their bodies require. Women naturally have lower levels of a neurotransmitter called serotonin, and this important "feel good" chemical drops even lower during menstrual cycles. In order to raise levels of serotonin rapidly, women tend to eat carbohydrates, which boost blood sugar, resulting in a rise of serotonin levels. Though carbohydrates do rapidly raise serotonin levels, once the blood sugar goes up and an insulin response occurs, the serotonin levels crash again, as I will explain in detail in Chapter Three. In order to limit their daily caloric intake, women tend to exclude protein in favor of carbohydrates, many of which have high glycemic indexes, that is, the body can rapidly convert them into sugar—such as pasta, potatoes, bagels, and so on. These carbohydrates are also directly responsible for loss of skin tone and increased body fat. Yet, with a proper diet composed of adequate protein, low glycemic carbohydrates, and the all-important essential fatty acids, serotonin levels can be elevated to much higher levels. Such a diet sustains these higher levels, keeping mood elevated and eliminating the continual craving for the unhealthy carbohydrates.

As I examined Jill, I found that her skin was very thin, almost translucent. She appeared to have very little sun damage, thanks to her scrupulous avoidance of sun exposure in hopes of preventing wrinkling. Nonetheless, as Jill was about to learn, sun exposure is just one cause of wrinkles, albeit a serious one. Her bone structure was excellent and she had the facial symmetry that is typical of a professional model. Yet overlying this perfect bone structure was skin that was very wrinkled, particularly around the mouth and the chin, where the skin had taken on a crinkled look caused, I knew, by inflammation. This crepeyness is indicative of long-term inadequate nutrition, a signature of marginal protein intake, and it cannot be corrected in just three days. However, I knew that the appearance of this crepeyness would improve after the Three-Day Nutritional Face-lift, and that the long-term program would greatly diminish the accumulated damage.

I felt that I could turn Jill around. If she would follow the anti-inflammatory diet during the upcoming three-day weekend, I promised her she would be rejuvenated by Tuesday morning—a person who both looked and felt renewed. I also gave Jill a topical amino acid formula that was placed in a transdermal delivery system. This formula had demonstrated great success in restoring libido.

Jill was skeptical that a simple change in the way she ate could make much difference in her appearance, or that a lotion could restore her libido. She was soon to learn that our food choices have everything to do with how we look and affect wrinkles, skin tone, eye bags and puffiness, and facial vibrancy and clarity.

The wrinkle-free eating plan is high in anti-inflammatory antioxidants. My diet eliminates all foods that cause a proinflammatory, or proaging, response. Have you ever taken a good look at yourself the morning after you've eaten Chinese takeout? The pasty, puffy face staring back at you is the direct result of an inflammatory response to what you ate. Just as the wrong foods can age you—right before your eyes—the right foods can take years away in as little as three days. Of course, the longer and more faithfully you follow the full 28-Day Wrinkle-Free Program, the younger and healthier you will look and feel.

The Core Wrinkle-Free Eating Plan

This is the generic eating plan, the same protocol I give all my patients. Each day, you must consume:

- Eight to ten glasses of water
- Three meals, evenly spaced throughout the day (always eat protein first)
- Two snacks, one mid-afternoon and one between dinner and bedtime (again, protein first). Each meal and snack must contain one of my recommended sources of protein, carbohydrate, and fat in the form of omega-3 and omega-6 essential fatty acids.

At this point, there is no need for you to know the science behind why you are eating the foods I recommend and how they will rejuvenate you. Remember: this is a test run. I will give you a specific menu for three days of eating. There is no guesswork involved in the Three-Day Nutritional Face-lift.

A Second Chance

Four days after her initial visit, Jill returned for a checkup. She was animated and excited and claimed that she just couldn't have imagined the difference that three days of eating could make. Jill's energy level had risen. By day two of the plan, her mood and demeanor were upbeat and optimistic. By day three, she barely recognized the vibrant, cheerful, energetic stranger smiling back at her in the mirror.

Jill's skin had begun to take on a porcelain-like luster, and her pores were noticeably smaller. Her cheekbones seemed higher, her brows lifted, and the hollows in her face more contoured. The skin around her mouth that had been crepey and wrinkled was visibly smoother. Jill's entire face had taken on a look of refined elegance.

Her biggest challenge during the three days had been to overcome her fear of eating three meals and two snacks per day. Jill, like many women, hadn't eaten that much food in one day since she was a teenager.

Many women avoid drinking water for fear of bloating, a complete misconception. The great majority of us are in a constant state of dehydration—drinking water only when we experience thirst, which is too little too late. All biochemical reactions take place in the presence of water. If we are even just mildly dehydrated, metabolism drops by 3 percent, resulting in a one pound weight gain every six months. It is essential to drink eight to ten glasses of water a day. If you have any doubts about the effect of water intake on your skin, just put a grape and a raisin side by side.

Jill's adherence to the regimen had produced the desired changes. I knew that if Jill continued with the 28-Day Wrinkle-Free Program the results would be even more dramatic. Much of the damage that she had believed could only be corrected with Botox, surgery, or chemical peels would repair itself with the full program, which also includes supplements, topical skin care products, and exercise.

"I feel as if I've been given a second chance—a new lease on life," Jill said. "I don't know what is more thrilling for me—the way I look or the way I feel. I only know that there's no going back to my old habits." Jill also reported that the topical libido enhancer had worked wonders.

Without exception, every patient who has tried the Three-Day Nutritional Face-lift has had good results and has returned convinced that my Wrinkle-Free Program works. And you will, too.

Before You Begin

Now, you can endure practically anything for three days, but you will find that the Three-Day Nutritional Face-lift is neither a chore nor an ordeal. Of course, you will want to select a three-day period during which you can control what you eat. Obviously, you will not want to start during the holidays or while you are on vacation. Though you can "eat the wrinkle-free way" at any time in any place, most of my patients find it easiest to start the regimen during a quiet weekend.

Planning is always an important part of following any program. Make sure you have what you need on hand or plan to shop each day to ensure you are eating the freshest food available. Following the menus, I will provide a shopping list to make preparation for your three-day test run efficient and easy.

In order to achieve optimal results, the three-day diet is more radical than the 28-day program. It is extremely important to eat *two portions of salmon a day*. I do not recommend smoked salmon for the three-day diet, as it tends to be salty. You may substitute canned salmon (mixed with a tiny bit of mayonnaise or with fresh lemon juice) for grilled salmon, but not more than once a day.

Eat only what is on the menu. It is critical that coffee is completely eliminated from our diet. Coffee raises levels of cortisol and insulin, hormones that accelerate aging and store body fat. Substitute green tea instead, which contains catechin polyphenols, antioxidants that boost metabolism and slow aging. Green tea can also block the absorption of bad fats by 30 percent, while the amino acid theonine promotes a sense of calm and improves one's mood. And, of course, avoid chemical-laden diet sodas.

Everything you need to eat to boost your energy and become radiant from the inside out is in the Three-Day Nutritional Face-lift. Get ready for your transformation!

The Three-Day Menu

You will be eating close to the same thing each day. Remember to *always eat your protein first.* Though this diet has some variety, a restricted diet is often easier to handle since you are not confronted by too many choices.

Wake Up
- 8 to 12 ounces spring water

Breakfast
- Omelet made of 3 egg whites and 1 yolk and/or a 4- to 6-ounce piece of grilled or broiled salmon
- ½ cup cooked oatmeal (not instant)
- 3-inch slice cantaloupe and ¼ cup of fresh berries (blueberries, if possible)
- 8 to 12 ounces spring water (minimum, more if desired)

Lunch
- 4 to 6 ounces grilled salmon or low-sodium canned tuna packed in spring water or sardines packed in olive oil
- 2 cups romaine lettuce; dress with 1 tablespoon extravirgin olive oil and freshly squeezed lemon juice to taste
- 3-inch slice cantaloupe and ¼ cup of fresh berries
- 8 to 12 ounces spring water (minimum, more if desired)

Mid-afternoon snack
- 2 ounces low-salt, sliced chicken breast
- 4 raw, unsalted hazelnuts
- ½ green apple
- 8 to 12 ounces spring water (minimum, more if desired)

Dinner
- 4 to 6 ounces grilled salmon
- 2 cups romaine lettuce; dress with 1 tablespoon olive oil and freshly squeezed lemon juice to taste

- 1 cup steamed asparagus, broccoli, or spinach dressed with a little olive oil
- 3-inch slice cantaloupe and ¼ cup fresh berries
- 8 to 12 ounces spring water (minimum, more if desired)

Before-bedtime snack

- 2 ounces low-fat low-salt turkey or chicken breast
- ½ pear or green apple
- 3 or 4 almonds or olives
- 8 to 12 ounces of spring water (minimum, more if desired, but bear in mind this is before bed)

This menu calls for six 8- to 12-ounce servings of water. Beyond that, you should drink at least two additional glasses throughout the day. Keep fresh water on your desk at work, a bottle of water with you in your car, or close at hand at home to sip as you are doing chores or cooking, to stay well hydrated.

That's it. What could be simpler? These meals and snacks require minimal preparation, which will keep you out of the kitchen and away from temptation.

The Shopping List

Here's all you need to prepare for your three-day diet:

· Dozen fresh eggs

· Oatmeal (*not* instant). Instant oatmeal will rapidly raise your blood sugar, cause a burst of inflammation, and ruin the results. Old-fashioned oatmeal is slowly absorbed by the body.

· A minimum of 1½ to 1¾ pounds fresh salmon cut into six portions

· 8 ounces thinly sliced low-salt turkey or chicken breast

· 1 can sardines packed in olive oil (if you chose this option for lunch)

- · 1 can of low-sodium tuna packed in water (if you chose this option for lunch)
- · 2 ripe cantaloupes
- · 1 pound asparagus
- · 1 pound broccoli
- · 1 pound fresh spinach
- · 2 heads romaine lettuce
- · 1 pint strawberries
- · 1 pint blueberries
- · ½ pint raspberries
- · ½ pint blackberries
- · 3 green apples (e.g., Granny Smith)
- · 2 pears (or an additional 2 green apples)
- · 2 lemons
- · Olives of any type—fresh or canned
- · Raw, unsalted almonds
- · Hazelnuts
- · macadamia nuts
- · 8-ounce bottle extravirgin olive oil
- · 3 or 4 gallons spring water

The Payoff

The more closely you stick to this diet, the better results you will achieve. After three days, you should be well on your way to controlling inflammation and fluid retention, and as a result your skin will glow and your energy soar.

In order to realize quick results, the foods allowed on the Three-Day Nutritional Face-lift are limited. The food choices in the 28-Day Wrinkle-Free Program are far less restrictive, and it is a way of eating you can live with forever. But whenever you need a special lift, you can return to the Three-Day plan to cleanse your system and rejuvenate your spirits.

Consider the Three-Day plan a secret weapon, a spa in a diet. You can be assured that you will always look and feel your best by following this simple eating plan.

I know it takes a leap of faith to follow this plan blindly, but I am certain it will be worth your while. I will explain the theories behind my Wrinkle-Free Program in the balance of the book, so you will understand the remarkable age-fighting attributes of the food you eat. In the following chapter, you will learn how inflammation causes aging . . . and how to reverse its relentless progress.

2

The Inflammation-Aging Connection

Though the correlation between inflammation and aging has only recently been recognized, I have spent my entire medical career studying this connection and searching for ways to prevent it. Today, research, academia, industry, and medicine all accept the causal relationship between inflammation and most chronic degenerative diseases, an astonishing list that includes arthritis, multiple sclerosis, atherosclerosis, diabetes, Alzheimer's disease, osteoporosis, asthma, cirrhosis of the liver, bowel disorders, meningitis, cystic fibrosis, cancer, stroke, psoriasis, and, of course, aging.

This chapter explores the inflammation-aging connection on a cellular level and demonstrates how wrinkles happen. After reading these pages and learning how free radicals operate, you will never again want to expose your skin to the sun without serious protection. But that is just one situation we have learned to control. My mission has been to discover other ways to avoid hidden, gradual cellular damage. In order to protect yourself, you need to understand the process of aging.

Making the Connection

By the time I entered medical school, I had already served in the army and had been the director of the Muscular Dystrophy Association. Perhaps it was those few extra years in the "real world" that made me less overwhelmed, less accepting of conventional wisdom, and thus more questioning than my fellow students. I was always eager to shake things up, to challenge traditional thinking.

One distinct advantage I had over the others was my ardent interest in nutrition. When I was discharged from the army, I left the fatigues behind but not the fatigue. I was mentally and physically exhausted and also suffered from allergies. In my search for help, I read Linus Pauling's books and was intrigued by his theories about vitamin C and the common cold. I also read the work of Adele Davis, a popular—if a bit radical—nutritionist in the 1960s and '70s. I was convinced that supplements would help my condition and began taking them. As I experimented with various nutritional supplements, I started to feel more energetic.

I then turned to exercise and its benefits to overall health. Regular exercise helped me build muscle and become more physically fit. I found that I was not only more productive but also more enthusiastic about my work and daily life. My allergies abated. My cognitive function and concentration improved greatly. I was surprised—and thrilled—to experience such dramatic changes.

I incorporated my personal experience into my medical studies. During patient rounds I would often ask myself "How could this process be therapeutically altered with nutritional supplements?" When I studied a disease process, I was inspired to find new therapies that would complement traditional treatments. I discovered that I was interpreting what I was seeing in a different manner from my colleagues. My unique approach has enabled me to develop a number of revolutionary breakthroughs in the treatment of aging and aging skin.

During medical school and my three-year residency in dermatology, I made some important connections between inflammation and disease. In addition to learning about the hundreds of skin diseases through book study, we had to be able to recognize them on clinical examination of patients and identify them under a microscope. This is called the "histopathological correlation" to the clinical examination. In other words, first we look at the disease in real life, and then we examine the tissues under the microscope. This allows us to understand on a microscopic level what is causing the clinical appearance seen by the naked eye. When studying various forms of skin cancer, I noticed that every time I saw a skin cancer under the microscope, inflammation was present at the cellular level. I questioned my professors, and their explanation was that the body mounts an immune response to try to fight the cancer, resulting in inflammation. I asked them if there could be more to it than that, since the inflammation was present even when the cancer was not full-blown, as I had observed inflammation with pre-cancers under the microscope. I asked my professors if an inflammatory response could be *triggering* or *promoting* cancer. But they persisted with the explanation that the inflammation is an immune *response.*

Medical students are quick to learn that discretion is the better part of valor, and topics like this are not open for debate. Nor does a medical student's opinion have much weight. Regardless, I just couldn't accept that answer. It wasn't just cancer and pre-cancer that showed inflammation under the microscope. When I looked at a biopsy of skin that showed clinical signs of aging, inflammation was present. Yet skin that showed no clinical signs of aging showed no inflammation. This discovery so intrigued me that I began to search for ways to put my emerging theory to the test.

In order to examine inflammation under the microscope, the slide containing the specimen must first be stained so the inflammation, if present, will be visible. Inflammation has unmistakable characteristics, and shows up as little dark-blue dots, almost like confetti—although the presence of inflammation is nothing to celebrate. Quite the opposite is true. This "confetti" is present whenever we examine aging skin. I was puzzled about why this inflammatory response was occurring. I wondered if inflammation was actually causing these changes in the skin. I began to consider wrinkles a disease, since inflammation was always present when damage to skin tissue resulted in wrinkles. I was driven by a number of questions. Were the negative signs of aging just a normal, unavoidable fact of life? Or were they an abnormal condition caused by an inflammatory state? Could many of the visible effects of aging be greatly reduced—or avoided altogether?

My professors thought inflammation was merely a part of the whole picture, a by-product and not the cause. For example, it was pointed out, your thumb turns red and swollen (by-product) after you accidentally hit it with a hammer (cause). And yet, ironically, one of the cornerstones of dermatologic therapy is cortisone, which is, of course, an anti-inflammatory. The tongue-in-cheek description of dermatological practice is that if you see a skin disease, and it is wet, you dry it; if it is dry, you wet it; and if you don't know what it is, you treat it with steroids (cortisones), which are powerful anti-inflammatories. I could not understand why the medical establishment refused to make the connection.

I knew what I saw and never let it go. I continued to believe that inflammation was at the root of cancer and other acute and chronic diseases. Whenever I looked at a disease under a microscope—everything from arthritis to heart disease—inflammation was always a component. Every disease I studied had a common theme, whether it was cancer or aging: inflammation was present. I was convinced that inflammation was not simply a secondary response. I believed inflammation to be the key to the whole process of disease of every type.

This powerful conviction led me to develop an inflammation-aging theory and inflammation-cancer theory that has been the basis of my research for decades. I realized that regardless of where a disease originated, regardless of its cause, anti-inflammatories often solved the problem, or at least diminished the symptoms. Cortisol does come with the high price of serious and often dangerous side effects. Although cortisol might be indicated in certain dermatological conditions, their anti-inflammatory properties are not traditionally recommended for most diseases. Since I believed that inflammation was the basis of disease, my goal was to find anti-inflammatories that could stop, treat, and reverse the symptoms without doing harm.

Naturally, my first step as a dermatologist was to search for ways to control inflammation in the skin. Every skin problem or disease I saw had an inflammatory component to it. Our skin is constantly assaulted from inside and out by elements that create inflammation: sun exposure, air pollution, harsh soaps and skin care products, internal disease, stress, lack of sleep, sugar consumption, dehydration—the list goes on. At the top of that list are sugar and foods that rapidly convert to sugar, known as *high-glycemic carbohydrates* ("bad" carbs). (Sugar's effects are discussed in the next chapter.) My research has focused on disarming these threats to healthy skin. The program I have developed is designed to fight inflammation by means of a synergy of diet, supplements, skin care, and exercise. To understand why my recommendations work, you have to know the mechanics of inflammation and its connection to aging and disease.

Why We Age

The free radical theory is the most widely accepted theory of aging. Free radicals are at the root of many acute and chronic diseases as well. On a cellular level, they are responsible for severe damage.

The atoms and molecules that make up our bodies have one or more pairs of electrons in their outer orbits. In the 1950s, Denham Harman, M.D., Ph.D., identified free radicals as atoms or molecules that are missing one of their two electrons, thus compelling the free radical molecules to complete their structures. When a molecule or atom is missing one of its electrons, it is unstable and will try to take another electron from any other molecule in its immediate environment. If a free radical acquires an electron from the molecule next to it, then that molecule or atom may become a free radical. In turn, the new free radical attacks a molecule next to it. And so on. Thus, we have a chain reaction of molecules that are desperately seeking completion, leaving severe damage in their wake; for each time an electron pair is broken, damage occurs to the victim molecule. Denham Harman postulated that it is the damage to these molecules that leads to aging. The medical community essentially ignored Harman's theory for twenty years. It was not until scientists finally started finding evidence of the importance of free radical chemistry in biologic aging systems that his theories began to gain acceptance.

Thanks to Dr. Harman, we learned that free radicals are troublemakers. You may be wondering where they come from. Free radicals are mostly derived from oxygen, the molecules of which tend to lose an electron, becoming unstable. These solo molecules are called "reactive oxygen species." Obviously, we need oxygen to live; it is part of the air we breathe, and it enables our bodies to metabolize food into energy. At the same time, oxygen becomes dangerous when it loses an electron and becomes a free radical, or a reactive oxygen species. By understanding the process, we can defeat it.

The Formation of Free Radicals

The conversion of food to energy in our bodies is accomplished in or-ganelles; tiny structures within our cells called mitochondria. The mito-chondria may be thought of as "little furnaces" that take food that has been broken down into its basic chemical structure and then combine these chemicals with oxygen, producing water and energy. The problem is that about 5 percent of the energy produced turns into reactive oxygen species. The chemical reactions in the mitochondria are one source of free radicals. In addition, free radicals are created in very high levels throughout the body whenever there is trauma, infection, or inflamma-tion. When we walk outside on a sunny day, the sunlight immediately be-gins to trigger free radical formation in our skin, which causes damage to our skin and to the tissue beneath it. I will describe this process in detail later in the chapter.

We live in an oxygen-rich environment. Fortunately, nature has built-in defense mechanisms against free radicals. These defense systems are called antioxidants, which prevent damage from oxygen. You are no doubt familiar with many antioxidants, like vitamin C, vitamin E, and beta-carotene, all of which we derive from our diet. Our body creates en-dogenous antioxidant systems as well. Some of these are enzyme systems and others are amino acids, like glutathione, which can stop free radicals in their tracks. Glutathione, composed of three amino acids, controls the antioxidant status of our cell (more about this antioxidant later). Let's look at a free radical rampage more closely.

Guarding the Gate

Envision one of your cells as a castle. Inside the cell are important com-ponents such as DNA and the mitochondria that are necessary for health,

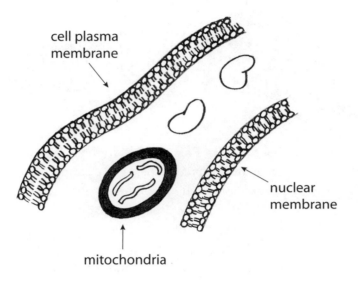

cell plasma membrane

nuclear membrane

mitochondria

reproduction, and life itself. As a castle is surrounded by a moat, the cell is encased by the cell plasma membrane that is filled with fat. The cell plasma membrane is a lipid bilayer: two thin layers of fat sandwiched together. The cell plasma membrane, like a medieval moat, surrounds the cell and protects it from invasion by enemies. It does more than just encase the vital inside of the cell (known as the cytosol). The cell plasma membrane is covered with receptors for hormones and neurotransmitters that enable our bodies to function.

For a long time, most scientists believed that the cytosol (core of the cell), which contains the vital machinery of the cell, was the site of the majority of free radical damage. But Dr. Imre Nagy, a Hungarian scientist, disagreed. He contended that the free radicals were doing the heaviest damage on the outside of the cell, in the cell plasma membrane. His theory is known as the membrane hypothesis of aging. Nagy claimed that free radicals are able to do so much damage in the cell plasma membrane because it is a molecularly dense area. Simply put, the cell plasma membrane has a high concentration of material vulnerable to damage. Therefore, he concluded, the cell plasma membrane is the critical first line of

cell plasma membrane

defense in protecting the cells. Free radicals do their damage by random hits; they are unstable and unpredictable. For example, if a tennis ball bounces around a room containing just a few chairs, there is not much damage that ball can do. If, however, the room is fully furnished and the tennis ball bounces around, it will knock over a lamp or shatter Aunt Sally's teacup collection. Damage will be done. Since the cell plasma membrane consists of a dense concentration of molecules, free radicals are bound to cause damage.

The cell plasma membrane must remain fluid to function properly. As we age, the membrane stiffens and loses its fluidity. When the membrane becomes inflexible, nutrients can no longer *penetrate* the cell. Conversely, when thick and stiff, the membrane can no longer pass waste *from* the cell. The wastes build up and cause our enzyme systems to slow down until we are unable even to replicate DNA or RNA. When the cell membrane loses fluidity, receptor sites for hormones and neurotransmitters cannot function. And this is how the cell ages.

Nagy realized that we had to protect the cell plasma membrane if we want to prevent cellular damage from free radicals. Since antioxidants are the cell's free radical defense system, Nagy outlined the criteria for antioxidants to be effective:

1. The antioxidant has to have greater affinity for the free radicals than the tissue. In other words the antioxidant has to be able to scoop up the free radical before it can damage the cell.
2. The antioxidant must be nontoxic. Just because a substance functions as an antioxidant in a test tube does not necessarily mean that it will work in the body.

3. The antioxidant has to be able to get to the site where protection is needed.

The cell plasma membrane is a fatty environment composed of two layers of phospholipids (see below for a complete definition). In order for the antioxidant to penetrate this fatty shield, it must be fat soluble. In addition, this fat-soluble antioxidant must be powerful enough to inactivate the free radical before it does damage to the cell plasma membrane. As you can see, it is critical that a therapy possess the correct molecular structure to protect us from the ravages of inflammation and aging.

The Scientific Secret to Youth and Beauty

My research has taken the findings of Drs. Harman and Nagy a step further. My divergence from the earlier membrane hypothesis uncovered a new characteristic of the cell plasma membrane. Though the cell plasma membrane is a free radical shield, it is also the source of inflammatory chemicals that wreak havoc if they get inside the cell.

As mentioned earlier, the cell plasma membrane is made up of two layers of phospholipids. The phosphate portion may be thought of as the head, and the lipid portion as the tail. The fat-soluble portion (the tail) of the phospholipid molecule points inward; and the water-soluble portion (the head) points outward. This results in a stable bilayer, because we find water both outside the cell and within the cell interior.

When free radicals are generated by ultraviolet radiation—for example, during a walk in the sun—those free radicals live for just a nanosecond. As a result, they do very little *direct* damage. But these short-lived free radicals trigger the phospholipids in the cell plasma membrane to break down into toxic inflammatory chemicals. These chemicals can then leak into the interior of the cell.

When the phospholipids break down, they produce a fatty acid, called arachidonic acid, and oxidized fats. Some of these oxidized fats convert to aldehydes, toxic chemicals, triggering an inflammatory cascade. Let's examine the process.

phospholipid

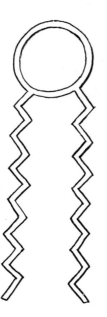

We know that the lipid bilayers of the cell membrane have eight times more oxygen than other parts of the cell, and that oxygen dissolves in fats. The high level of oxygen in the cell membrane creates the ideal environment for producing oxygen-based free radicals. And it is the oxygen-based free radicals that are the most abundant and most damaging to our bodies. So, when we walk outside and the sunlight strikes our skin, generating oxygen-based free radicals, these free radicals are very reactive and attack the phospholipids. During the brief life of the free radical, the phospholipids are oxidized and changed into toxic oxidized fats. These toxic fats, some of which are converted to aldehydes, flow into the cell and cause damage to the interior of the cell and to the DNA.

It Gets Worse

This oxidized fat can mimic important chemicals in the body, including platelet-activating factor, which controls inflammation. Platelet-activating factor can initiate inflammation. The oxidized fat attaches to the same receptor as the platelet-activating factor would, fooling the body and generating an inflammatory cascade that damages blood cells and arteries and places us at risk for deadly blood clots.

Arachidonic acid is a fatty acid that is released by the cell plasma membrane when inflammation (or free radicals) attacks the cell plasma membrane. Arachidonic acid is then broken down into proinflammatory chemicals such as prostaglandins, which may cause PMS symptoms, including swelling, bloating, depression, etc. When arachidonic acid, produced by the breakdown of phospholipids by free radical attack, invades the mitochondria, it interferes with energy production, disrupting our metabolism. Instead of food being converted to energy, in the form of ATP (a high-energy phosphate that provides energy in our cells), the energy is released in an uncontrolled manner that causes the generation of more free radicals. Those free radicals then do damage to the mitochondria, further aging our skin.

Enzyme systems oxidize the arachidonic acid into a number of proinflammatory chemicals, including prostaglandins and leukotrienes, and HETES. The inside of the cell is extremely sensitive to inflammation, and these proinflammatory chemicals cause a good deal of damage. Remember the chain reaction: whenever inflammation is present, more free radicals are triggered, resulting in damage to the cell and accelerated aging. The process is threefold and cyclical:

1. A burst of free radicals attacks the cell plasma membrane.
2. The cell plasma membrane produces proinflammatory chemicals.
3. These proinflammatory chemicals produce *more* free radicals.

The Survival Factor

The cell has defenses of its own, which I think of as the "survival factor." Antioxidants are the cell's defense against oxidants (free radicals). The cell monitors the ratio of oxidants (the bad guys) to antioxidants (the good guys). We call this ratio "the redox level."

Here's what happens on a cellular level. Redox-sensitive indicators report redox level changes, and the cell responds defensively. Next, glutathione, a tripeptide made up of three amino acids, comes into action. Glutathione is important in cell defense against free radicals and oxidative stress, and it regulates the chemical balance of the cell. Whenever a cell is under severe oxidative stress, glutathione comes to the rescue, but it gets used up quickly and its levels drop. In fact, a low glutathione level is an almost perfect indication of chronic and acute inflammatory states. Luckily, we are now able to increase and maintain high levels of glutathione to maximize our cellular defenses. I will discuss strategies for doing so later.

The Birth of a Wrinkle

The interior of the cell is filled with a gelatinous material that houses the nucleus, DNA, and protein "transcription factors." These proteins are nothing more than tiny molecular messengers that can move to the nucleus to stimulate our DNA to replicate RNA and make important proteins for cell function. Here we want to concentrate on two important transcription factors, nuclear factor kappa B (NF-kB) and activator protein 1 (AP-1). These transcription factors are not active in the cell unless the redox level of the cell changes and free radicals are about to overwhelm the cell's defense mechanism, a state called oxidative stress. When the cells undergo oxidative stress, the transcription factors are activated. NF-kB migrates to the nucleus and attaches to the DNA, resulting in cellular production of proinflammatory cytokines—chemicals that are the so-called "serial killers" of the cellular world. AP-1 migrates to the nucleus where it causes the production of a variety of chemicals, including collagenases, which digest collagen. Our beautiful, youthful skin, chiefly composed of collagen, has no defense against these collagen-digesting enzymes. When collagen is digested, it results in the microscars that lead to wrinkles.

The Fountain of Youth

You should now have a good picture of the inflammation-aging connection. All the devastating cell damage I have described is triggered by just one thing—inflammation. It would logically follow that anti-inflammatories are the answer. I thought that if I could find a chemical that would act as an antioxidant anti-inflammatory in the cell plasma membrane, I could prevent much of the damage I was observing. I had to find powerful antioxidant anti-inflammatory molecules that were fat soluble so they could protect the cell plasma membrane *and* prevent the cascade of events that lead to premature aging and a host of degenerative diseases.

As the following chapters will reveal, I have discovered a strategy that reduces oxidative stress throughout the cell. By protecting the cell plasma membrane, the lipid bilayers that surround critical portions of the cells, inflammation can be minimized, preventing accelerated aging. By using such nutritional powerhouses as salmon, extra virgin olive oil, and a host of antioxidant supplements, we can fight against the ravages of time on our faces and bodies. Simple physical exercises also help us in the battle.

If you follow my program, you will take control of the rate at which you age. *The Perricone Prescription* is as much about learning what not to do as it is about learning what to do. Just as your choices can keep you young and rejuvenate your physical and mental states to a degree you never dreamed possible, so too can your choices accelerate the aging process. This knowledge can change your entire life, as it has for me and many of my patients and students. You can be healthy and active well into your eighties. You can start a new career at seventy. You can take up new hobbies late in life. Your cognitive function can be at its peak when you are sixty-five or seventy. An entirely new, tremendously rich stage of life is opening up for all of us. So read on to make the right choices in nourishing your body as you begin your journey toward being wrinkle-free for life!

3

The Wrinkle-Free Diet

My patients are always surprised when I tell them there is only one obstacle that stands in their way to looking and feeling young. Of course, they want me to tell them what it is. I hand them a mirror.

Once you accept that your everyday lifestyle choices affect the way you age, you are on your way toward restoring your youthful looks and vigor. Nutrition is a major weapon in the battle against inflammation. What you eat fuels your body and sustains the extraordinary complex systems that keep you alive. The Perricone Wrinkle-Free Program takes into account everything your body needs to stay healthy and strong. The Wrinkle-Free Diet will show you the best choices to make for maximum health that will be reflected in every aspect of your life.

I frequently wonder how it can be possible, in the midst of so much plenty, that the majority of us deny our bodies and brains the nutrients we need to fight aging. Few of us are seriously underweight, we appear well nourished, and yet most of us are beggars at life's banquet. You must provide your brain with the nutrients it needs to function at peak levels, to solve problems, to keep memory sharp, to generate creative ideas, and to experience a state of well-being. Your body needs a steady supply of high-quality protein and the right fats. What your body does not need is sugar and high-glycemic carbohydrates, like rice, pasta, and potatoes. Sugar and foods that are rapidly converted to sugar are potent inflammatory agents and, consequently, among your skin's greatest enemies.

The failure to eat adequate, high-quality protein results in the breakdown of your cells and the body's inability to repair them. This damage is unnecessary and 100 percent avoidable. In place of the protein we need, we often consume large quantities of foods that rapidly convert to sugar in our bloodstream, causing an immediate inflammatory response. And by now you know: inflammation equals aging. Inflammation is the reason you get wrinkles, why you forget everything from where you left the car keys to your neighbor's first name, why you can be irritable and depressed, and why you lose the healthy bloom of youth.

Many of you will automatically recoil at the thought of eating fats, mistakenly thinking fat makes you fat. Our culture's aversion to and rampant fear of fat is dangerous. Essential fatty acids are critical for the healthy function of cells. As a physician, I have seen the ravages of the low-fat, no-fat diet craze, and they are alarming. Your body needs to be a well-oiled machine. Later in this chapter, you will meet Jack, who suffered the seriously detrimental effects of a low-fat diet.

With the Perricone Wrinkle-Free Diet, you will learn the difference between fat that kills and fat that is the key to a long healthy life. If you starve your cells of essential fatty acids, which are needed to fuel the mitochondria, your body cannot burn up and metabolize the fat you consume. Instead, that fat is stockpiled as extra padding on your thighs, buttocks, upper arms, and abdomen. And so we keep trying every fad diet that comes along.

The purpose of this chapter is to give you the background you need to make the right nutritional decisions day in and day out. When you know how sugar triggers inflammation, when you picture the chain reaction ruining your health, you will find it easier to resist that chocolate chip cookie or bowl of pasta. When you realize that protein is essential to cellular repair, that it supplies all of the essential amino acids needed for life, you will want to shift the balance of what you eat, sidestepping carbohydrates for the best protein choice—fish. An understanding of how essential fatty acids and monounsaturated olive oil promote radiant good health will assure you that these are fats to be welcomed in your diet, not avoided. This knowledge has made a big difference in the lives of my patients. Let me tell you about Megan.

Megan and the All-American Continental Breakfast

When I first met Megan, she was about twenty pounds overweight, lethargic, and experienced bouts of depression. She was frequently sick, catching every cold, flu, or stomach virus that went around. Of Italian-Irish lineage, she had an olive complexion. Her skin was loose, jowly, and large pored. She tended to have dark circles under her eyes no matter how much sleep she got.

Megan had just quit her dead-end job and, at the age of thirty-five, enrolled in graduate school. She wanted to turn her life around, beginning with a diet and liposuction.

Megan, like all of us, wanted to look good, enjoy a positive and upbeat mood, perform mental tasks at the highest possible level, and have plenty of energy and motivation to stay physically fit. Very few of us score a ten in any of these areas, and Megan was no exception. Yet none of these goals was out of her reach. She just needed to relearn everything she thought she knew about what to eat.

Believe it or not, it is not simply genetics that determines cognitive ability, great skin, athletic prowess, and temperament. Yes, genetics plays a part, but the rest is determined by biochemistry. And here is where you can learn to influence the hormonal and chemical responses in your brain and body. Food is the key.

Food is much more than just a life-giving and life-sustaining substance—it is our single most powerful antiaging tool. The choices we make daily—or even hourly—directly influence our physical and mental states, the number of wrinkles and amount of sagging in our faces, our overall muscle and body tone, the condition of our internal organs, our brain and memory power, and our mental and emotional states. The vast range of available fats, proteins, and carbohydrates that comprise the modern diet represents an entire pharmacological cornucopia.

Although Megan wanted to begin her transformation with liposuction, I preferred to get her started on the right foods to rebuild her body and allow it to function in an optimal manner. In addition, I knew that the right foods would help ensure that her bouts of depression did not recur.

Since food works in your body like a drug, it can bring you up or drag you down, scramble your brain or accelerate your cognitive skills, increase hyperactivity or induce extreme fatigue. Food can keep you awake or put you to sleep. Food influences every automatic body function, from your ability to burn fat to the regulation of your hormones.

I asked Megan what she had for breakfast, and she proudly described a breakfast eaten daily by millions of men and women. She faithfully followed what she considered a healthful, low-fat diet and started each day with:

- A large glass of orange juice
- A bowl of cereal (raisin bran or cornflakes) topped with sliced bananas
- Skim milk
- Low-fat bran muffin
- Pat of no-cholesterol margarine
- Cup of coffee

Here is what this "healthy" breakfast is doing to Megan. As she drinks the juice, she is causing a burst of inflammation in her body, as the juice floods her bloodstream with sugar. This causes a sharp spike in her insulin levels, resulting in a rapid acceleration of the aging process, increasing the risk of heart disease, every form of cancer, memory loss, and mental deterioration. To add to the problems, the sugar flood is causing the collagen in her skin to cross-link, laying the foundation for the birth of wrinkles, sagging, and loss of tone. The coffee increases her insulin level further and also stimulates cortisol, the stress hormone, which causes the abdomen to store fat and is also toxic to brain cells.

And the juice is just the beginning. Now Megan turns to the cereal, banana, and muffin, all of which rapidly convert to sugar in her bloodstream and dangerously raise insulin levels. The cereal and bananas are equivalent to eating as much sugar as you would find in a Snickers candy bar. But the Snickers bar is less inflammatory, because it contains fat. Fat retards the absorption of sugar, thus slowing down the production of insulin. Since there is no fat in the skim milk or muffin, there is nothing to decelerate the carbs from rapidly converting to sugar, causing an insulin spike. This typical low-fat breakfast will store body fat more quickly than eating the candy bar! It is also grossly deficient in the protein necessary for total body repair. The absence of good fats can cause diverse problems, such as mental depression, heart disease, and dry skin.

After you have eaten such a meal, your "feel good" brain chemical serotonin will drop dramatically so that you will not only be fat, wrinkled, and fatigued, you will also be in a bad mood. And if you are suffering from PMS, you can be assured that this meal will magnify your symptoms. At this point, let's discuss how sugar creates and aggravates inflammation.

Sugar, Inflammation, and Aging

Sugar and high-glycemic carbohydrates—fruits and vegetables that rapidly convert to sugar—create inflammation on a cellular level throughout your body. If you eat a large quantity of refined sugar or a bowl of pasta that converts to sugar in the bloodstream, the sugar triggers an insulin response from the pancreas to control the level of blood sugar in your body. Diabetics do not have a properly functioning pancreas, and consequently they suffer from high blood sugar, which must be treated with insulin. Diabetics with poorly controlled blood sugar actually age one third faster than do nondiabetics. Diabetics tend to have widespread, measurable inflammation in their bodies. Their constant high sugar levels cause kidney failure, blindness, heart attacks, and strokes. Studies have shown that when diabetics keep their blood sugar levels within normal range, they can cut their rate of health problems by 70 percent.

Elevated blood sugar causes a number of chemical reactions in the body that create inflammation. For starters, blood sugar reacts with minerals in our body, such as iron and copper, creating free radicals, which then attack the lipid bilayer membranes of our cells. This results in a cascade of proinflammatory chemicals, causing further damage and accelerated aging.

Sugar causes inflammation in several ways. When blood sugar goes up, it creates free radicals that oxidize fats. And as you learned in the previous chapter, oxidized fats are bad news. Our cholesterol can also become oxidized. We know there are two kinds of cholesterol, LDL and HDL. LDL is supposed to be the bad cholesterol, HDL the good. In reality, LDL cholesterol is not bad unless it becomes oxidized. High blood sugar causes LDL to oxidize. When oxidized, it encourages plaque deposits in our arterial lining. These deposits cause the blood vessels to clog, leading to coronary artery disease.

Even though a diet high in saturated fats such as beef, pork, lamb, and full-fat dairy products was believed to lead to heart disease, that is not entirely accurate. These foods are only part of the story, and not necessarily the largest part. A diet high in pasta, cereals, breads, rice, rice cakes, potatoes, sweets, desserts, and juices can actually lead to heart disease. In other words, the bun may be worse than the burger. Ideally, you will avoid both. Diabetics have a higher incidence of coronary artery disease than nondiabetics do, probably because their high blood sugar is causing LDL to oxidize.

Carbohydrates and the Fat Production Paradox

Americans have also been sold a bill of goods about which carbohydrates to eat and which to avoid. Our focus on meat and potatoes, dairy products, refined carbohydrates, and sugar addiction has made us the leaders in cancer, stroke, and heart problems. We can also lay claim to being the most overweight nation on the globe.

Whenever sugar increases insulin levels in the body, fats are also stored. This leads to obesity, even though caloric intake may not necessarily be excessive. A rice cake has about 45 calories and 0 grams of fat. Yet this dietary mainstay of millions of American women can make you fat. Rice cakes are quickly converted to sugar, because puffed rice has a very high glycemic index, making it proinflammatory. Eating a rice cake

Remember this irrefutable fact:

insulin release = stored body fat

will generate the insulin response that causes us to store rather than burn fat.

Glycation, Cross-Linking, and Leathery Skin

You don't have to be diabetic to experience an inflammatory response from sugar. Even a healthy body is damaged by sugar in a phenomenon known as glycation. When foods rapidly convert to sugar in the bloodstream, as high-glycemic carbohydrates do, they cause browning, or glycating of the protein in your tissues. Glycation is a process long known to discolor and toughen food in storage. Glycation can occur in skin as well, creating detrimental age-related changes to collagen—and that means deep wrinkles.

When glycation occurs in your skin, the sugar molecules attach themselves to the collagen fibers, where they trigger a series of spontaneous chemical reactions. These reactions culminate in the formation and gradual accumulation of irreversible cross-links between adjoining collagen molecules. This extensive cross-linking of collagen causes the loss of skin elasticity. Healthy collagen strands normally slide over one another, which keeps skin elastic. If a young person smiles or frowns, creating lines in the face, the skin will snap back and be smooth again when she stops smiling or frowning. But the skin of a person whose collagen has been cross-linked from years of eating carbs and sugars does not snap back and smooth out. Those deep grooves remain, because that is where the sugar molecules have attached to collagen, making the fibers stiff and inflexible.

The bond between the sugar and collagen generates a large number of free radicals leading to more inflammation. When glycation occurs in the skin, the ultimate effect is not unlike tanning a hide. Over time, skin begins to resemble a cross between beef jerky and an old boot, unevenly discolored and heavily striated with deep lines and grooves.

Besides being visible in our faces, we can easily see the aging properties of carbohydrates in the laboratory. Fibroblasts are the cells that produce collagen and elastin fibers, the strands of tissue that give skin its strength and flexibility. If just a drop of sugar is added to a cell culture of fibroblasts, within a minute or two we can measure a sharp rise of inflammatory chemicals in the cells. I should add that glycation takes place in all parts of the body and can destroy other vital organs, including your kidneys, lungs, and brain.

Sugar can also attach to components in the cell plasma membrane forming chemicals called advanced glycosylation end products, appropriately known as AGES. Accumulation of AGES in a cell can lead to malfunction and, as the acronym indicates, aging. As my research revealed the effects of sugar on the skin, sweets and starches permanently lost their appeal for me.

The Rating Game—The Glycemic Index

The glycemic index is one of the keys to looking and feeling younger than your years. This simple tool is a helpful road map through the maze of seductive foods beckoning from supermarket aisles and restaurant menus. This scale rates foods according to their impact on blood sugar levels.

The glycemic index I use rates foods on a scale of 1 to 100, with 100 indicating the increase in blood sugar levels resulting from eating table sugar. The 28-Day Perricone Program excludes those foods with a glycemic index above 50. For example, plain yogurt has a glycemic index of 14, which is acceptable. By comparison, white French bread has a glycemic index of 95, meaning it is quickly digested and will flood the bloodstream with glucose. A "healthy" breakfast bar comes in at 87, and good old-fashioned rolled barley packs a wallop at 100!

There are two versions of the glycemic index—one based on sugar (glucose) equaling 100, and one based on white bread equaling 100. Each is a good indicator of the relative value of various foods. I prefer to use the sugar-based list and the numbers in this chapter reflect that preference. For the most up-to-date information regarding the glycemic index ratings for the foods you eat, go to http://www.mendosa.com/gi.htm.

Glycemic Horrors

These are foods that should be avoided at all costs. The glycemic index ranks how foods affect your blood sugar levels. The index measures how much your blood sugar increases in the two or three hours after eating. The rankings for this list and all others that appear in this chapter are based on glucose as 100.

Tofu frozen dessert (nondairy)	115
French baguette	95
Gluten-free bread	95
Instant rice	90
Rice Chex cereal	89
Hamburger bun	87
Rice cakes	82
Cornflakes	82
Rice Krispies	82
Pretzels	81
Vanilla wafers	77
Doughnut	76
Waffle	76
Corn chips	73
Bagel	72
LifeSavers candy	70
Croissant	67
Angel food cake	67

You can be carrying five thousand extra calories on your thighs, but you will not be able to burn it off, because the insulin in your bloodstream creates a "lock," which means that those calories cannot be accessed for fuel. If you want to get rid of those five thousand calories and let your body live off that fat, don't eat anything with a glycemic index over 50. Otherwise, the insulin surge caused by high-glycemic foods will guarantee that your body fat stays firmly "locked" in place, regardless of how few calories or fat grams that food contains.

Antioxidant Best Bets

Avocado
Bell peppers
Berries
Cantaloupe and honeydew melons
Dark green leafy vegetables (spinach and kale)
Orange-colored squash
Salmon
Tomatoes

Though it is obvious that you are not going to eat a sticky bun, think twice before you reach for a carrot, which is high in sugar. If you are interested in a broader approach to the subject, I suggest you read *The Zone* by Dr. Barry Sears, who helped pioneer the acceptance of the glycemic index in controlling blood sugar, losing weight, and improving performance.

Carbohydrates—The Good, the Bad, and the Ugly

Simple sugars—including table sugar, honey, molasses, and maple syrup—must be relegated to fond memories. You know the kind I mean: those fond memories of tooth decay, acne breakouts, and weight gain. These foods have no nutritional value and create an immediate inflammatory cascade in your cells. If you want to retain your youthful appearance and keep your muscles and joints functioning at optimum levels, avoid these foods completely.

Foods to Avoid

Alcoholic beverages (including aperitifs, hard liquor, wine, beer, and liqueurs)
Bacon
Bananas
Breads
Bagels
Beef
Butter
Carrots
Cream cheese
Candy
Cake
Chocolate
Coffee
Cookies
Cereals (except noninstant oatmeal)
Cornstarch
Corn, corn syrup
Croissants
Dried fruit
Duck
Doughnuts
Fruit juice
Fried foods
Flour
Grapes
Granola
Half and half
Hard cheese (*except* feta, Parmesan, and Romano)
Heavy cream
Honey
Hot dogs
Ice cream
Jams and jellies
Mango
Margarine
Molasses
Muffins
Noodles
Oranges
Pancakes
Papaya
Pastry
Peas
Pie
Pizza
Pasta
Pickles
Popcorn
Potatoes
Pudding
Pumpkin
Raisins
Relish
Rice
Sherbet
Soda (including diet)
Scones
Sugar
Tacos
Waffles
Watermelon
Whole milk

Complex carbohydrates like corn, pasta, rice, and bread do contain nutrients, including iron, calcium, fiber, and B vitamins, but with few exceptions they cause more problems than benefits. As a group, they can trigger a rapid rise in blood sugars and create a fat lock in the body, preventing us from being able to burn or utilize our body fat for energy. On the Wrinkle-Free Diet, I limit carbohydrates found in grains, and include only whole grain, noninstant oatmeal, and legumes like lentils and beans. These foods are absorbed slowly and will not provoke an inflammatory reaction from a surge in blood sugar levels. To stay young, we need to have a slow, steady release of insulin into our bloodstreams.

Portion size is another factor you must keep in mind to keep blood sugar levels stable and thus prevent inflammatory reactions in the body. Even anti-inflammatory foods can provoke an insulin response if we eat too much at one sitting, and carbohydrate intake especially must be monitored. In the Wrinkle-Free Diet, I limit each serving of lentils, beans, or oatmeal to no more than ½ cup per meal, as larger portions at a single meal will set off an inflammatory cycle.

The 28-Day Perricone Program does not mean a lifetime without ever having pizza, pasta, or bread. Once the diet is an established part of your lifestyle, you can have one of these foods once a week. Your body can handle some of these foods if you understand the balance. For example, if you eat a pasta dish, make sure to eat your protein first. Choose high-fiber whole-wheat (9 grams of fiber per serving) pasta, and cook it al dente (firm). Then serve it tossed in olive oil, freshly chopped parsley, and lightly sautéed garlic, garnished with Italian grating cheese such as Parmesan. The fiber and olive oil slow the absorption of the carbs in the pasta, as does the al dente preparation. The antioxidants and minerals in the garlic and parsley complete the picture. But always remember to eat the protein first, and follow with the pasta and salad. And be sure to eat a small serving of pasta—no more than two ounces uncooked. If you eat pizza, limit yourself to one slice.

The Good Carbohydrates

The body must have carbohydrates to function. To meet these nutritional needs, my diet includes four to seven servings of low-glycemic carbohydrates in the form of fruits and vegetables. As a group, these foods are packed with vitamins, minerals, and antioxidants to slow or reverse signs of aging while supplying essential energy. They also contain water, which helps hydrate the skin and body. Choose fresh or frozen produce, but avoid canned items, as heating and processing destroys many nutrients while adding unwanted salt and sugar.

Foods to Enjoy

Almonds	Chicken (white meat)
Apples	Chilean sea bass
Asparagus	Clams
Avocado	Cod
Beans (black, kidney, lima)	Coriander
Bell peppers (green, orange, purple, red, yellow)	Cottage cheese, low-fat
	Crab meat
	Cucumbers
Blackberries	Dill
Blueberries	Egg whites
Broccoli	Eggplant
Broccoli rabe	Endive
Brussels sprouts	Escarole
Cabbage	Low-fat milk
Cantaloupe	Fennel
Capon	Feta cheese
Cauliflower	Filet of sole
Celery	Flounder
	Garlic

Ginger (fresh)
Grapefruit
Halibut
Hazelnuts
Honeydew melon
Kale
Kiwi
Leafy greens
Legumes
Lemons
Lentil soup
Lettuce
Lobster
Monkfish
Mushrooms
Mussels
Nectarines
Nuts
Oatmeal (not instant)
Olive oil
Olives
Onions (red and white)
Parmesan cheese
Parsley
Peaches
Pears

Pecans
Plums
Radishes
Raspberries
Salmon
Sardines
Scallions
Scallops
Shrimp
Smoked salmon
Snow peas
Sour cream
Soybeans
Spinach
Swiss chard
Swordfish
Tea
Tofu
Tomatoes
Tomato juice
Trout
Turkey
Walnuts
Yogurt
Zucchini

Avoid dried fruits.   They are calorie dense and are concentrated balls of fructose, a form of sugar. Although fructose does not cause an insulin response, it can still attach to collagen, forming the glycation reaction.

A number of popular fruits and vegetables have a very high glycemic index, so be vigilant. Only beets rate higher on the glycemic index than carrots, that mainstay of so many low-calorie diets. Carrots have a high glycemic index, higher than cookies or ice cream. Yet carrots have vitamins and fiber, so they possess redeeming qualities that cookies do not.

Wrinkle-Free Fruits	Less Desirable Fruits
Cherries	Dates
Grapefruit	Watermelon
Pear	Pineapple
Apple	Raisins
Plum	Apricots
Peach	Mango
Orange	Banana

Please do not think that if a junk food has a lower glycemic index than a fruit or vegetable you might be justified in eating it. If the choice is between a brownie and a banana, choose the fruit—at least it has vitamins and fiber. Keep in mind that the glycemic index is a rough indication, because when you take foods in combination, their absorption rates alter and change the index.

Cooking and juicing make a difference, too. For example, carrots rate higher on the glycemic index if you cook or juice them. So, if you eat a carrot, have it raw. If you follow my plan, you will avoid any confusion about food choices. Everything I recommend that you eat is under 50 on the glycemic index.

Are You Convinced Yet?

All that damage from o.j., a muffin, cornflakes with bananas? Pasta and garlic bread? A soft drink and potato chips? All this and much more. Remember: when we eat excessive amounts of sugars or carbohydrates that are converted quickly to sugar, our body produces insulin in a frantic attempt to lower our blood sugar. Eventually, the insulin receptors on the surface of the cells no longer function properly—they burn out. Our blood sugar rises along with insulin levels, which leads to excess body fat.

Food acts like a drug. If we eat the right food, it protects us from proinflammatory chemicals being produced by free radicals. The next time you sit down to a high-carbohydrate meal with high-glycemic foods, remember, it may feel good for a few moments, but you are starting an inflammatory fire in all the vital organs of your body, including your skin, which will show these proinflammatory effects.

> ### Veggies to leave on your plate:
>
> | | |
> |---|---|
> | Parsnips | Beets |
> | Baked potato | Corn |
> | Fava beans | Sweet potato |
> | Pumpkin | Cooked carrots |

In your daily food selection, you unconsciously choose foods that exert a druglike effect on your moods, emotions, and physical state. This is why we use terms like "addicted to carbs," "sugar junkie," "junk food addict," or "sugar high." The problem lies in the "high," because what goes up must come down—and the crash is not much fun, whether it's from sugar or caffeine. Our mood drops even lower than it was before the fix of a bagel; cookie; or caffeinated, sugary soda. So we eat or drink more of the same, exhausting our pancreas, burning out our adrenals, and placing us at risk for insulin resistance and diabetes.

For the balance of this chapter, I want to focus on what you need to eat to lose body fat, raise your energy, erase wrinkles and stop new ones from forming, increase skin elasticity and muscle tone, and elevate your overall feeling of well-being. Let's start with protein.

Of First Importance

Protein is the basic material of life. In fact, the word "protein" comes from an ancient Greek root meaning "primary" or "first." The body could not grow or function without it. Since the human body can manufacture only twelve of the twenty-two amino acids that are essential for life, the remaining nine must be provided by eating food. However, the contemporary American diet rarely contains protein in sufficient quantity to maintain and repair cell and skin health.

If I were to poll my patients and students about what food they crave, I can assure you the answer would never be a grilled salmon filet. Most of my patients tell me their first choice when hunger strikes is a latte and brioche or a rice cake and diet soda. At a fast-food restaurant, their usual order consists of French fries and a salad with nonfat dressing—and their faces show it. Sadly, an ongoing lack of protein is first noticeable in the face, as the features become soft and doughy. The sharp definition, contoured cheekbones, and that great jawline all become blurred. When the protein supply is depleted, the body is forced to feed upon itself. This causes both tissue and muscle to break down.

Once you know what to look for, you can immediately spot a person who eats a high-carb, low-protein diet. You can see it in women and men as early as their twenties. So remember, the lack of protein in your diet translates into highly visible changes in your face and body—and these changes are not improvements. The first critical step is to ensure that you consume adequate protein throughout the day.

The Inside Story on Good Looks—How Protein Works

In my efforts to find answers to why we age, I reasoned that if aging and aging skin are characterized by the breakdown of our cells, the antidote to aging might be cellular repair. Protein is essential to cellular repair. The building blocks of our cells are composed of amino acids. As protein is digested, it breaks down into amino acids that are then used by the cells to repair themselves. Without adequate protein, our bodies enter into an accelerated aging mode. Our muscles, organs, bones, cartilage, skin, and the antibodies that guard us from disease are all made of protein. Even the enzymes that facilitate all-important chemical reactions in our body—from digestion to building cells—are made of protein. This simple fact of life can change the way you look beginning with your next meal. If your cells do not have complete availability of all the essential amino acids, cellular repair will not only be incomplete but also will be much slower than it should be.

In my practice, I have often seen chronic, low-grade, long-term protein starvation lead to a loss of face and body skin tone in many of my female patients. Their breasts start to sag and show early signs of stretch marks. Within a matter of weeks of starting a diet rich in high-quality protein (especially that found in fish like salmon), the skin starts to firm up on the face and body, and there is a visible lifting and improvement in skin tone and texture.

Research indicates that women need at least 65 grams of protein daily. Adequate intake for men ranges from 75 to 80 grams. The final figure depends on height, weight, and level of physical activity. This protein requirement is easily met with just ten to fourteen ounces of high-quality protein each day. Notice I specified *high-quality* protein.

> **Remember this key fact:** we cannot store protein in our bodies. If you want to keep your face and body firm, toned, lithe, and supple, you need to provide it with a fresh supply of high-quality protein every day. That's three meals a day and two snacks.

As with fats and carbohydrates, all forms of protein are not equal. When I refer to protein, I mean animal protein. Although vegetarian diets rely on protein derived from combinations of various grains, vegetables, and legumes to provide the necessary amino acids, it is still not high-quality protein. I have also found that servings of these concentrated carbohydrates cause metabolic problems that override their potential health benefits.

For example, a single serving of grilled chicken breast delivers 28 grams of protein at 172 calories. The protein content of ½ cup of cooked rice ranges from 2 to 2.5 grams and contains 103 calories. You would need to eat seven cups of rice—packing a whopping 721 calories—to get the same amount of protein as in the chicken breast. To add insult to injury, the amino acid profile is not complete in rice. A half-cup serving of navy beans has 7 grams of protein and 110 calories. You would have to eat two cups of beans to get 28 grams of protein—440 calories—and the beans also do not provide a complete amino acid profile. Beans are an important source of carbohydrates and fiber, but I recommend no more than ½ cup per meal.

This mixing and matching of proteins is a lot of work, and many vegetarians have problems getting enough protein, high quality or otherwise. Then there is the effect of this volume of carbohydrates on the body. You know what eating starchy foods like potatoes, rice, and corn does to the collagen fibers in the skin. Diets heavy in carbohydrates create a highly visible inflammatory effect on the face and body. This is particularly apparent in my vegetarian patients, who often appear years older than they actually are. Their skin sags more, and their skin color tends to be dull rather than rosy. They are often more moody, cranky, and tire more easily than my patients who follow my eating plan.

Best Protein Choices

Although I recommend animal protein, I do so with some reservations. Certain protein choices can create a proinflammatory response, which equals accelerated aging. I believe that previous research condemning saturated fats due to their correlation with cardiovascular and other diseases is somewhat erroneous. The saturated fats found in full-fat dairy products and red meats (including beef, veal, lamb, and pork) can be proinflammatory in large amounts (due to arachadonic acid content), and thus portion size should be limited. Instead, opt for fish, egg whites, skinless chicken and turkey breast.

All You Need Is Fish

Of all the foods that can keep you young, fish tops the list. All fish is an outstanding source of high-quality and easily digested protein with low saturated fat. What makes fish stand out from other excellent protein sources is its type of fat and fatty acid content, both of which have powerful anti-inflammatory effects.

> · Seafood is nutrient dense. That means it offers large quantities of protein and significant amounts of vitamins and minerals without high levels of saturated fats and calories.
> · Seafood is an excellent source of complete protein, providing all the essential amino acids. The protein in seafood is easily

digested, making it a perfect nutrition source for people of all ages.

· Seafood is a good source of B vitamins and provides key minerals and trace elements such as calcium, magnesium, potassium, phosphorus, sulfur, fluorine, selenium, copper, zinc, and iodine—elements necessary for proper development and growth.

· Seafood contains a very small amount of fat. The fats that it does contain are "good fats." Most varieties of fish and shellfish contain less than 5 percent fat. Even high-fat fish generally have less than 15 percent fat, which is considerably lower than the amount in red meat. Seafood is also lower in saturated fat than most other protein sources. By substituting fish for meat in some of your meals, you can considerably lower your total fat and saturated fat intake.

· Seafood is generally low in sodium. Most fresh fish contain very low amounts of sodium, ranging from 60 to 100 milligrams per 100 grams, or 3½ ounces of raw fish.

· Cholesterol levels are not significant in most seafood—and looking at cholesterol alone can be deceptive. Although fish are generally quite low in cholesterol, shellfish has low to moderate amounts. Even species with high cholesterol levels, like squid, contain less cholesterol than eggs, and are well within the 300 milligram daily limit recommended by leading health organizations.

(SOURCE: "Seafood for the Good Life . . . A Basic Introduction to Seafood Nutrition," National Fisheries Education and Research Foundation)

Protein should be present at every meal and every snack to provide energy and means of cellular repair throughout the day. When you start my program, weigh your protein servings for every meal. Within a few days, you will be able to judge by eye the correct portion size. Patients on my anti-aging diet often start out eating fish two to three times a week.

When they see how fast their skin improves, they are quick to increase their fish intake to five to seven meals each week. You should plan to eat a seafood meal seven days a week—and salmon at least five times a week. You can choose fresh, frozen, canned, or smoked fish.

Make sure salmon is your first choice. You can buy Alaskan red or pink salmon in the can. It tastes wonderful with just a little lemon juice squeezed on it and takes all of sixty seconds to prepare. Canned salmon is wild salmon, not farm raised. Whatever fish or shellfish you choose, sauté, grill, poach, or broil it, brushing it lightly with olive oil. For additional antioxidant protection, season with garlic, onions, lemon juice, and tomatoes.

Beauty and Brains

The flesh of fish—especially salmon—contains DMAE, a powerful antioxidant. This chemical stimulates nerve function and the muscles to contract and tighten under the skin. DMAE is your magic bullet for great skin tone, keeping your face firm and contoured. It prevents and reverses what is clinically known as "anatomical loss of position," commonly known as sagging.

Only one food has the reputation from time immemorial of being a "brain food." That food is fish, especially fish that is high in DMAE. DMAE is recognized as a cognitive enhancer. A diet high in DMAE will enable you to think more clearly, improve your memory, and increase your problem-solving ability. DMAE is a building block of the neurotransmitter acetylcholine. Like other neurotransmitters, acetylcholine allows one nerve to communicate with another, or to communicate with a muscle. Studies have also shown that DMAE acts as an antioxidant by stabilizing cell membranes, protecting them from free radical damage. By raising levels of DMAE in our bodies, we can think more clearly and have greater muscle tone in both face and body.

Once you decide to move any muscle in your body—whether to type on the computer or curve your lips into a smile—a signal emanates from the brain and travels along a nerve until it approaches the appropriate muscle that will do the actual job. At the end of the nerve is a bud that holds a reservoir of neural chemicals including acetylcholine. The nerves do not actually touch the muscle to make it jump into action. Instead, the signal stops a short distance away at a place known as the "neuromuscular junction," just before contact. Here, the powerful neurotransmitter acetylcholine is released from the bulb and locks onto special receptors on the muscle, causing the muscle to contract. As we age, our levels of acetylcholine decline, resulting in reduced muscle tone. Instead of staying short and tight, the muscles become elongated and relaxed, resulting in a sagging face and body.

You will improve muscle tone if you increase your acetylcholine levels, and one of the best ways to do this is by introducing additional DMAE into your system. The four steps that work synergistically to provide optimum levels of DMAE in the body are:

1. Eat fish, the only significant dietary source of DMAE.
2. Take DMAE in the form of a nutritional supplement.
3. Apply a high-potency, rapidly penetrating DMAE topical lotion to the skin on the face and body.
4. Keep the muscles toned with exercise.

The chapters that follow will cover points 2, 3, and 4, all integral parts of the 28-Day Wrinkle-Free Program. Point 1 is up to you!

I believe that the improved muscle tone that results from the Three-Day Nutritional Face-lift is due in great part to the rise in acetylcholine levels from the daily servings of salmon.

Fats to Plump up the Skin

The Perricone Wrinkle-Free Diet is *not* a fat-free diet. Fat-free diets are a one-way ticket to trouble. Fats and oils provide essential anti-inflammatory and antioxidant protection. Though it is true that certain saturated fats, like those found in red meat, are not ideal, but not prohibited, it is easy to learn what fats to eat every day and what fats to eat sparingly or avoid altogether. Fats have become such a taboo for the weight conscious, but you must understand how they work and how the right fats can help you lose weight.

How Fat Is Used in Your Body

1. Fats can be burned as fuel in the mitochondria but cannot be utilized for energy unless essential fatty acids are present.
2. Fats can be stored as body fat.
3. Fats can be incorporated into the cell membrane for good or ill. Good fats will have a stabilizing effect on the cell and will prevent breakdown into inflammatory chemicals.
4. Fats can act as hormone-like substances directing fat metabolism in the cell.

Chemically, fats and oils are made up of chains of carbon molecules edged with hydrogen and oxygen molecules. When the carbon chain is completely full of hydrogen, it is called a saturated fat (for example, butter and lard). When the chain is missing two hydrogen molecules, it is considered a monounsaturated fat. Olive oil is the best example of a monounsaturated fat. If the carbon chain is missing four or more hydrogen molecules, the fat is said to be polyunsaturated (for example, corn oil and fish oil). Monounsaturated and polyunsaturated fats are liquid at room temperature. Each type of fat has different properties and different effects on the body.

Saturated Fats

These fats, which are solid at room temperature, include vegetable fats, such as Crisco or shortening, and animal fats, such as butter and lard. High intake of saturated fats is linked to heart disease, increased blood pressure, stroke, diabetes, gallbladder problems, as well as breast and ovarian cancer. However, I believe that trans fatty acids are the worst offenders, which I will describe later in this chapter. Research has shown that the wrong types of saturated fats can have a strong inflammatory effect on the body. To avoid proinflammatory, proaging responses, you must limit your intake of red meat (beef, veal, pork, and lamb) to one serving per week.

Dr. Perricone's Body Fat Metabolizing Formula

Here is my fail-safe formula for whenever I need to lose body fat:
- CLA (conjugated lipoic acid)—1,000 mg three to four times a day
- ALA (alpha lipoic acid)—250 to 500 mg a day
- CoQ10 (coenzyme Q10)—60 to 120 mg a day
- acetyl L-carnitine—500 to 1,000 mg a day (take on an empty stomach)
- L-carnitine—500 mg three times a day
- DMAE—75 mg twice a day
- L-tyrosine—500 mg twice a day
- GLA (gamma linoleic acid)—1,000 mg a day
- Omega 3—500 mg twice a day (take one if you are eating fish)
- chromium polynicotinate—200 mcg per day

I have also found that after five years of working with patients on the anti-inflammatory diet that those who eat cold water fish daily—especially Alaskan salmon for breakfast—have found this greatly facilitates fat loss and appetite control.

Little Shop of Horrors—Trans Fats, or Polyunsaturated Fats

Polyunsaturated fats from vegetable sources, including corn oil, safflower oil, and canola oil, have been heralded for years as "health food" because of their ability to lower LDL (bad) cholesterol. Yet retrospective studies show an increased cardiovascular risk from diets high in polyunsaturated fats. Contrary to what you have been led to believe, you should avoid polyunsaturated fats.

When these fats are processed by chemically adding hydrogen to extend the shelf life of foods that contain them, they produce solid trans fatty acids. These are called "Franken-fats," and they are the most damaging fats of all. They do not occur naturally in nature. Trans fats are produced commercially to turn vegetable oils into shortening and margarine, making them solid at room temperature. Food manufacturers also use partially hydrogenated vegetable oil to destroy certain essential fatty acids, linolenic and linoleic acid in particular, that tend to oxidize and cause fat to become rancid. French fries and other fast foods are usually cooked in this kind of partially hydrogenated oil that contains trans fats. Commercial baked goods often contain trans fats to act as a preservative. None of this is for your benefit; it is for the benefit of the food manufacturers.

Trans fats present a genuine danger to health. There is another reason to avoid trans fats: they decrease insulin sensitivity by making the cell membrane stiff and inflexible. The best way to avoid these unnatural trans fatty acids is to stay away from processed foods and margarine. Learn to understand food labels. You'll be shocked to discover how many supermarket foods contain these dangerous fats. On the Wrinkle-Free Diet, you will not eat any foods that have trans fats, so you can protect yourself from these culinary horrors if you follow my accepted food lists scrupulously.

Killer Fat

According to the Harvard University Department of Nutrition, on November 12, 1999, the Food and Drug Administration announced its proposal to include the trans fatty acid (trans fat) content of foods on the standard food labels, because:

> The combined results of metabolic and epidemiologic studies strongly support an adverse effect of *trans* fat on risk of CHD. Furthermore, two independent methods of estimation indicate that the adverse effect of *trans* fat is stronger than that of saturated fat. By our most conservative estimate, replacement of partially hydrogenated fat in the U.S. diet with natural unhydrogenated vegetable oils would prevent approximately 30,000 premature coronary deaths per year, and epidemiologic evidence suggests this number is closer to 100,000 premature deaths annually. These reductions are higher than what could be achieved with realistic reductions in saturated fat intake.
>
> ("*Trans* Fatty Acids and Coronary Heart Disease." Arnold, Jill, Harvard University Department of Nutrition, November 15, 1999.)

This shocking finding should convince you that foods containing trans fats are to be avoided at all times. Believe me when I say they are ubiquitous. They are in everything from pancake mix to peanut butter.

The Fish Story—More Beauty-Brain Connection

Polyunsaturated fats derived from fish, as opposed to bottled vegetable oil, are quite another story. Okay, I know there are some people who do not like fish. And they think they can get all the essential fatty acids and other nutrients contained in fish if they take fish oil capsules. This is a misconception. Many nutritionists and experts have focused on a few essential fatty acids that have been identified as being critical to our health. I believe there are probably dozens of unidentified fatty acids in salmon, for example, that play a crucial role in optimum health and the deceleration of the aging process. Polyunsaturated fatty acids, like those found in salmon, play a crucial role in the bodily process in which dietary fats are our major cellular energy source. Polyunsaturated fats also control the passage of compounds into and out of our cells because these fats become part of the cell plasma membrane. In addition, these fats serve as powerful hormones on a cellular level. If you don't like fish, start experimenting gradually. Countless patients have changed their feelings once they came to understand the amazing health and beauty benefits of eating fish. They are now seafood lovers. Flaxseed oil, which is best derived by grinding flaxseeds and placing them into your favorite beverage, provides omega-3 fatty acids that are not of animal origin. However, remember that in order to do its work, flaxseed must be converted to an active form in the body by an enzyme called delta-6. This enzyme is found in lower levels in women, older people, those under stress, people with atopic dermatitis, and some people with essential hypertension.

What Is the Difference Between Wild and Farmed Salmon?

· Without additives, the flesh of farm-raised salmon would not have the familiar pink color but would be gray.

· "Atlantic" salmon is synonymous with farmed salmon. Despite its country of origin—Norway, Chile, or Canada, for example—Atlantic salmon is the predominant farmed species. Wild Atlantic salmon are nearly extinct in the United States and Canada and are unavailable commercially. In Alaska, wild salmon are abundant and fish farming is currently illegal. Therefore, "from Alaska" or "Alaskan" always means wild. If the salmon is not labeled "wild" or "Alaskan," it is probably farmed.

· If it is fresh during the winter, it's probably farmed. Most wild salmon are harvested and available fresh only during the spring, summer, and fall. Wild salmon is available during the winter only in fresh-frozen, canned, and smoked forms.

· If there are white lines of fat running through the flesh, it is almost surely farmed. Farmed salmon spend their lives in small, densely crowded pens where they are hand-fed a pellet diet. A wild salmon migrates thousands of miles through open ocean, hunting its food and avoiding predators. This makes wild fish leaner. They display little or no visible fat.

What makes fish stand out from other excellent protein sources and makes it an extraordinary antiaging food is its multiple polyunsaturated fat and fatty acid content. Wild cold water fish—including salmon, mackerel, and trout—have the highest levels of omega-3 fatty acids. In their natural environments, these fish eat omega-3-rich plankton and later pass it on to us. The colder the water the higher the level of omega-3 in the plankton.

Shellfish is an excellent protein choice. However it does not have the essential fatty acids of fin fish, and its cholesterol content is a little higher. But I don't believe that cholesterol ingestion is a problem.

In general, the higher the fat content of the fish, the higher its omega-3 content—and the higher its antiaging brain and beauty benefits.

High-fat fish (more than 5 percent fat)
· Salmon
· Mackerel
· Albacore tuna
· Bluefin tuna
· Sablefish
· Sardines
· Herring
· Anchovies

continued on next page

- Shad
- Trout

Medium-fat fish (2.5 to 5 percent fat)
- Atlantic halibut
- Yellowfin tuna
- Mullet
- Swordfish
- Bluefish

Low-fat fish (less than 2.5 percent fat)
- Cod
- Pacific halibut
- Pollock
- Rockfish
- Shark
- Flounder
- Sole
- Croaker
- Grouper
- Red snapper
- Lingcod
- Sea bass
- Haddock
- Whiting

Essential Fatty Acids

Fat is one of the nutrients your body requires along with proteins, carbo-hydrates, and vitamins. The building blocks of fats and oils are called fatty acids. The fatty acids, known as essential fatty acids (EFAs), are those fats that we can't make in our bodies. We must obtain them from our food.

The essential fatty acids, like omega-3s and omega-6s, offer a wide range of health benefits. They are famous for their heart-protective effects and can lower blood pressure and decrease the chance of blood clots. In addition, studies have shown that even small amounts of fish in the diet can lower the risk of colon, breast, and prostate cancers. Doctors have found that the pain and inflammation of severe rheumatoid arthritis (another autoimmune disease on the rise and targeting women) is reduced by omega-3s. Laboratory studies of psoriasis patients indicate that they have low levels of omega-3. When treated with fish oil concentrates high in omega-3s, these patients find that their itchy, scaly patches improve. The omega-3 essential fatty acids dramatically reduce the body's production of inflammatory compounds. They actually block the production of arachidonic acid, a major cause of inflammation in the body. Omega-3 fatty acids are particularly good at targeting leukotrienes, chemicals that are provoked by the presence of free radicals and are known to promote allergies and skin disorders.

The omega-3 family of essential fatty acids are all derived from the molecule called alpha linolenic acid that is metabolized to eicosapentaenoic acid (EPA) and docosahexaenoic acid (DHA). These two omega-3 oils are found in high levels in salmon. It was once thought that most of the positive effects on the cardiovascular system were due to the EPA content of the essential fatty acids in fish. We have since discovered that the DHA portion is also extremely important to cardiovascular health. DHA has been shown to be more powerful than EPA in lowering triglycerides and increasing levels of the good cholesterol HDL. At the same time, DHA also has a marked effect in lowering blood pressure. But omega-3s are not the only essential fatty acids that have been shown to be beneficial to our cardiovascular health.

Sockeye Salmon (Oncorhynchus nerka), Red, Blueback

Wild Alaskan sockeye salmon are one of the most abundant and treasured of the wild Pacific salmon species. They have a deep red flesh and, of all wild salmon, have the highest concen-

continued on next page

tration of omega-3 essential fatty acids and the biological antioxidant astaxanthin. Studies suggest that astaxanthin is ten times more effective as an antioxidant than other carotenoids, and one hundred times more powerful than vitamin E. This natural pigment, which gives sockeye its rich color, comes from their diet of marine algae, zooplankton, and krill. Because sockeye live only about four years and eat primarily a vegetarian diet, they are less prone to accumulate harmful contaminants than are other species. EPA studies have shown Alaskan sockeye are among the purest fish ever tested.

Alaskan sockeye is available canned and, increasingly, fresh and frozen, as its unique characteristics have contributed to its growing popularity. When cooked or processed, the deep red flesh retains its color to a higher degree than that of other salmon. Sockeye is high in healthy fats, yet has firm flesh as well as a full, delectable flavor. The Alaskan sockeye's color, firmness, flavor, and nutritional profile make it one of the most desirable of all wild salmon species.

The omega-6 oils—found in borage oil and evening primrose oil to name a few key sources—are also valuable. Their active ingredients are derived from linoleic acid. One derivative of linoleic acid, GLA (gamma linoleic acid), has also been shown to have a positive effect on lowering cholesterol and triglyceride levels by increasing the good cholesterol HDL. To be sure you are getting the activated form of omega-6 oils (gamma linoleic acid), supplement your diet with borage or evening primrose oil. This is especially important as we age, as the levels of the activating enzyme delta-6 desaturase decrease as the years go by.

Both omega-6 and omega-3, in the proper 2-to-1 ratio, help to lower levels of "stress chemicals," such as cortisol and norepinephrine, which are elevated in the blood during stress. DHA significantly reduces norepinephrine levels in people who are chronically stressed. Further, as we age, our cortisol levels rise, making our cells resistant to the effects of insulin, resulting in increased body fat. When insulin continues to rise, blood sugar is not lowered. This state is known as insulin resistance, a condition that is often present in people who have elevated levels of blood fats and heart disease, and in those who have Type 2 diabetes. Research overwhelmingly indicates that GLA (from omega-6) and DHA (from omega-3) improve cell sensitivity to insulin and thus reduce our chances of developing heart disease, diabetes, and excess body fat.

Brain function is intimately tied to our essential fatty acid intake. Remember, essential fatty acids make up the phospholipid bilayer of the cell membrane. This is critical in the proper functioning of the nerve cells of our brains. There are high levels of DHA in human milk, and children who are nursed have optimal brain growth and development as infants. Deficiencies of DHA can lead to such problems as attention deficit hyperactivity disorder, which has become epidemic in this country; increased aggression; and a higher incidence of Alzheimer's disease later in life.

A final note—we have now discovered that essential fatty acids work via an extremely powerful mechanism on a cellular level. Essential fatty acids affect transcription factors in the nucleus of the cell, that regulate fatty acid metabolism. We have talked about other transcription factors; however, the transcription factors that are affected by essential fatty acids are called PPARs (peroxisome proliferator-activated receptors). These receptors activate certain portions of the gene that affect all aspects of fatty acid metabolism on a cellular level. The fatty acids derived from omega-6 (GLA) and those derived from omega-3 (DHA) activate factors that will alter gene expression. *Once again, we can see that portions of food, like essential fatty acids, can act like a powerful drug, affecting all aspects of our cells.*

If your diet is deficient in essential fatty acids, wounds cannot heal properly and you are more susceptible to infections. Your face and body become dehydrated—and you know what that does to your looks. Lack of essential fatty acids can cause sterility in men, miscarriages in women, arthritis-like problems, and some heart and circulatory problems.

Mood Menders

The most recent studies on omega-3 have linked low fish intake to an increased incidence of psychological problems, including depression, bipolar disorders, postpartum depression, and suicidal tendencies. In a study from Brigham and Women's Hospital in Boston, researchers found that patients with manic-depressive disorder who had not responded to conventional therapy improved dramatically when given a daily four-ounce serving of fresh salmon.

I have seen my own patients respond to "salmon therapy" with great success, and with no side effects other than younger, firmer skin, greater cognitive skills, and a lifting of the black cloud of depression.

Accutane

I occasionally prescribe Accutane, a powerful derivative of vitamin A, to treat severe cystic acne. Accutane is a "miracle drug" because it takes the worst, most deforming cases of acne and essentially renders a cure. Accutane achieves its miracle by altering fat metabolism on a cellular level, inducing a decrease in available fats, mimicking the effects of a low-fat or no-fat diet. Accutane has been reported in rare cases to cause severe mental depression. In order to help prevent this rare but serious side effect, I insist that my patients taking Accutane eat salmon daily. I also recommend essential fatty acids supplements in capsule form.

Most Americans—American women in particular—are critically deficient in these fatty acids and are aging rapidly and poorly as a consequence. These physical and psychological changes have been particularly dramatic in women who have spent years on a low-fat diet. When they come to me to deal with signs of aging, they are often already on medication to deal with anxiety or depression. As a physician, I know that psychopharmacological drugs are often necessary. However, these drugs all come with a price, and sometimes with serious side effects. Such side effects can include anything from weight gain to sexual dysfunction, from impaired memory to seizures. After twenty-eight days on the Perricone Wrinkle-Free Program, many of my patients discovered their emotional health had improved dramatically and, with the help of their physicians, they were able to reduce—and sometimes eliminate—their medications.

Megan's Rejuvenation

Megan responded extremely well to her new diet. After only six weeks, she confided that she had never felt more emotionally centered. Megan was also elated to discover that her skin actually glowed with health and radiance. For the first time since her teens, she had the energy and desire to exercise regularly. She was mentally and physically rejuvenated.

I had put her on topical antioxidants with DMAE for her face, and a high-potency body toning lotion for her thighs and upper arms. These, combined with her new exercise regimen, resulted in her body and her face fast becoming firm and toned; she was no longer considering liposuction! In addition, Megan was following a targeted supplement program, which I will explain in detail in Chapter Four. Megan now had the energy and self-esteem to start her new life with eager anticipation.

The Psychological Effects of a Low-Fat Diet

Women are not alone in suffering from mental depression and skin problems that can be successfully treated with dietary changes and targeted supplements. Jack, another patient of mine, is a case in point.

Twenty-seven-year-old Jack first appeared in my office complaining of a chronic rash. He had suffered from this rash for several years, and it was now worsening. He had been treating it with a variety of over-the-counter moisturizers with little success.

The rash was not his most serious problem. Jack had been suffering from severe mental depression and bipolar disease (manic depression) since his early twenties. He experienced frequent bouts of anxiety and insomnia. Jack was taking multiple medications, including antidepressants and lithium. As a result of his depression, Jack had been unable to complete college and drifted from one part-time job to another.

As I recorded his medical history, Jack explained that as a teenager he had been a competitive bodybuilder and had won many awards in his home state, Connecticut. At that point his depression and lethargy had not yet surfaced. Jack had been filled with energy, ambition, and expectations for a bright future.

I encouraged Jack to speak about this period of his life with me, as it seemed an excellent foundation on which to establish a relationship. I soon learned that as early as the age of fourteen, Jack began to alter his diet drastically. Bodybuilders, like fashion models, have been known to develop all sorts of bizarre eating habits. Just when he needed fat the most for normal adolescent growth, Jack cut all fats from his diet and ate only a carefully regulated high-protein, low-carbohydrate diet.

By the time he was eighteen, Jack began to experience bouts of depression and listlessness. His ability as well as his desire to compete in bodybuilding began to wane. No matter what dietary atrocity he committed—and there were many (eating only turkey breast and celery, for example)—he could not keep his body fat down. All the while, his depression continued to escalate.

The next part of his visit was a complete skin exam. I noticed that Jack had redness and scaling on many parts of his body. The diagnosis was atopic dermatitis, or as a more general term, what we refer to as eczema. Dermatitis is a fairly common condition, caused by a dysfunction in the immune system. Jack was surprised to learn that this type of eczema, with which he had struggled for years, could be improved simply by altering his diet and taking supplements. Jack was still avoiding eating fats; it was time to introduce him to the essential fatty acids.

I explained to Jack that a deficiency in essential fatty acids could lead to depression as well as skin problems. In addition, I explained that patients with atopic dermatitis sometimes had a deficiency of delta-6 desaturase and could not convert essential fatty acids in the active form, and I felt that his abnormal dietary restriction of fats over the years may have been responsible for many of his problems. I also explained that without the essential fatty acids, which are the building blocks of good prostaglandins, a malfunction of fat metabolism is certain.

Our first step was to start Jack on the anti-inflammatory diet. I strongly recommended that he begin eating fish, especially salmon, four to five times a week, if not daily. I also started Jack on a supplement regimen that included borage oil rich in GLA (gamma linoleic acid), the active form of omega-6. This complete supplement regimen will be explained in the next chapter. I gave him topical emollients containing polyenolphosphatidyl choline and a mild hydrocortisone cream for the more severe portions of his eczema.

Monounsaturated Fats

Monounsaturated fats that are solid at room temperature include animal fats, butter, and lard. There are also liquid monounsaturated fats found in olives, olive oil, and (to some extent) in nuts and avocados. Olive oil is such an important component of the Wrinkle-Free Program that it deserves its own discussion. Olive oil offers a wide range of health benefits. In addition to small amounts of vitamin E, olive oil contains both oleic acid and hydroxytyrosol. The same oleic acid that is found in the cell membranes of olive trees is essential for the cellular structure and functions of humans. Plants fill their seeds with fatty acids because they are the most efficient storage form of energy.

The Anti-Inflammatory Miracle of Olive Oil

Extra virgin olive oil is one of the most powerful anti-inflammatory foods in existence. Olive trees can live to be hundreds of years old, and they often rejuvenate themselves after being burned or even cut to the ground. Though I cannot promise you an equally long life span, I can assure you that you will look younger, think more clearly, be more active and, yes, extend your life if you incorporate extra virgin olive oil into your diet on a daily basis.

Olives and olive oil have been part of our history for thousands of years. As far back as 400 B.C., Socrates prescribed olive oil for curing ulcers, gallbladder problems, muscle aches, and a host of other conditions.

Fossilized olive leaves have been found that are one million years old. Olive trees were cultivated six thousand years ago during the Bronze Age in the Mediterranean basin.

A monounsaturated fat, olive oil is the type of fat that lowers LDL cholesterol at the same time it raises the level of HDL cholesterol. Extra virgin olive oil has the highest percentage of monounsaturated fat of any type of cooking or salad oil—including canola, peanut, corn, soybean, sunflower, and safflower—according to a study published in the *Journal of the American Medical Association*. Monounsaturated fats are very stable, because their molecule has only one reactive site. Olive oil does not have to be refrigerated, but should be stored in a dark, cool place.

Polyunsaturated fats, on the other hand, have many reactive sites, and easily oxidize to produce toxic lipid peroxides. If you have ever opened a bottle of vegetable oil that has been sitting in the cabinet for a period of months and have taken a whiff, you are familiar with the rancid odor of lipid peroxides. These chemicals are extremely toxic, even at very low levels. When ingested, lipid peroxides create massive inflammation in your body.

Not only oils can turn bad. Nuts, seeds, and grains can also become rancid, so store them in the refrigerator or freezer to be on the safe side. The fact is, you are actually poisoning yourself when you eat fats that contain lipid peroxide.

Although olive oil has only a small amount of the essential fatty acids, it contains about 75 percent of a nonessential monounsaturated fatty acid called oleic acid that helps to ensure that omega-3 fish oils penetrate the cell membrane. If you think of the cell plasma membrane as the door to the cell, then consider oleic acid as the key to that door.

Oleic acid is a member of the omega-9 family. In addition to enhancing the absorption of essential fatty acids, oleic acid can be incorporated into the cell plasma membrane to help maintain fluidity. Oleic acid helps to keep the membrane fluid, soft, and stable. It can make the difference between a complexion that resembles a piece of old shoe leather and one that looks and feels like a rose petal. In my search for powerful membrane stabilizers, oleic acid, as found in extra virgin olive oil, deserves a place at the top of the list.

The small amounts of essential fatty acids found in olive oil, along with oleic acid, perform a variety of anti-inflammatory miracles, an entire spectrum of services. For starters, a deficiency of linoleic acid can lead to eczema; hair loss; liver problems; kidney problems; and erratic, confused thinking. There is some very good evidence that olive oil can lower triglycerides, lower blood pressure, decrease the stickiness of platelets, and decrease heart attacks and their attending complications.

The Olive Oil–Cholesterol Connection

Another life-preserving fact about oleic acid is that it also decreases oxidation of LDLs (so called bad cholesterol). To visualize how LDL operates, think about rust. Rust occurs when metal oxidizes. Rust corrodes and eats away the metal, ultimately destroying it. Similarly, when LDLs are oxidized in our bodies by free radicals or sugar, the LDL molecules create an inflammatory cascade resulting in cell and artery damage, irritation of the artery walls, and fatty streaks. More oxidized LDL starts to build up at this spot, producing an artery-blocking plaque. Left untreated, this plaque eventually closes the artery entirely, leading to a possible heart attack or stroke. The anti-inflammatory antioxidants and fatty acids found in extra virgin olive oil provide a crucial defense against the oxidative effects that accompany aging, the human equivalent of rusting.

Olive Oil—A Panacea? Olé!

Studies continue to appear all over the world about the healing properties of extra virgin olive oil. Research conducted in Spain suggests that olive oil may help prevent colon cancer, an inflammatory condition. It should be noted that extra virgin Spanish olive oil contains the highest levels of a class of powerful antioxidants called polyphenols.

Studies from the Harvard School of Public Health suggest that women who ingest olive oil more than once a day have a 25 percent lower risk of breast cancer, another inflammatory condition. It is the proven role of olive oil in protecting the heart and cardiovascular system that brought attention to this disease-preventing, longevity-promoting food. In 1958, a longitudinal study, known as the Seven Countries Study, began and continued for more than fifteen years. The study looked at coronary heart disease and death from heart attack in the United States, Finland, the Netherlands, Japan, Greece, Italy, and Yugoslavia. The results made history: Greece and Italy had the lowest death rate from heart disease and the United States had the highest.

The difference? Olive oil! Greeks and Italians tend to eat a diet rich in the monounsaturated fat found in olive oil. This is in stark contrast to the typical American diet, which is literally swimming in trans-saturated fats and the low-fat diet of the Japanese. Although the U. S. Department of Agriculture advises Americans to "use all fats and oils sparingly," it does not differentiate among the kind of oils and fats we consume. It is telling that olive oil is used in the healthier Mediterranean diet on a daily basis. It is also important to note that obesity is rare in these countries yet rampant in the United States.

Some of the benefits of a diet rich in extra virgin olive oil:
- Increases the skin's ability to maintain moisture
- Evens out color, increases radiance when applied topically
- Decreases LDL (cholesterol)
- Increases HDL (cholesterol)
- Helps intestinal absorption of nutrients
- Helps gallbladder activity
- Lowers blood pressure
- Decreases gastric acid secretion in ulcers
- Lowers the probability of gallstones
- Stimulates pancreas secretion
- Aids bone development in children
- Prevents osteoporosis
- Lowers glucose levels in diabetics
- Reduces risk of prostate cancer
- Reduces risk of breast cancer
- Prevents edema (water retention)
- Prevents tumor promotion
- Beneficial to diabetes

But Wait—There's More!

We have discussed the fatty portion of olive oil, the oleic acid, but there are actually two elements in olive oil. The oily portion is known as the saponifiable fraction, which makes up the largest part of olive oil. But there is also a very small part called the nonsaponifiable fraction, and that contains such important components as beta-carotene and the olive oil polyphenols, which are very powerful protective antioxidants. One of the polyphenols, perhaps the most powerful, is hydroxytyrosol, found only in extra virgin olive oil. In addition to being a rare protective antioxidant, hydroxytyrosol is what gives the beautiful flavor to extra virgin olive oil.

Hydroxytyrosol is found in highest concentrations only in extra virgin olive oil that is obtained from olives grown in the Mediterranean region, particularly Spain. We don't know why this is. It might be the soil; it might be the particular type of tree. Even though hydroxytyrosol is found only in a few parts per million in olive oil, it is so powerful that it is probably the chief antioxidant in olive oil. Hydroxytyrosol slows the aging process in the skin by stabilizing the cell plasma membrane. Since it also prevents the oxidation of keratin protein, hydroxytyrosol makes the hair soft, shiny, and lustrous, and it prevents nails from peeling and breaking. And these great benefits can be yours with a daily salad of mixed dark leafy greens, topped with extra virgin olive oil.

Rating Olive Oils

Right about now, after reading about the myriad benefits of olive oil, you are probably ready to dive into a vat of it. But before you head for the market, you should know how to select the most healthful olive oil available. Where an olive oil is produced is only one factor to be considered when selecting olive oil for your kitchen and table. I recommend Mediterranean olive oil, because of the all-important hydroxytyrosol content. The ripeness of the olives at harvest time is also an important criterion.

When the olives are picked green early in the harvest season, the oils will be rich and fruity. If the olives have been left to ripen to a dark purple and harvested later in the season, the oil will be lighter and more mild flavored. The best oils are cold pressed between large millstones, just as they have been for thousands of years.

Producers run their mills continuously throughout the picking season when the olives are at their peak. If the olives are not pressed immediately they will oxidize, which affects the flavor and rating. The oil can only be called virgin olive oil if the oil is extracted by means of pressure from the millstones. They are not treated with heat or chemicals when the oil is extracted. Virgin olive oil is the oily juice of the fruit, and it must be processed at a particular time and in a particular way to maintain the distinctive flavor and aroma.

Batches of olives are pressed more than once to produce numerous batches, or "pressings," of olive oil. Olive oils are rated in the order of their pressing. The first pressing has the most desirable flavor and the lowest acidity, and this is the one I strongly recommend. At the second, third, and fourth pressings, the levels of acidity increases—and the price drops. With each pressing, the levels nonsaponifiable fractions drop, and the oils lose their antioxidant strength as the concentration decreases. The first cold-pressed olive oil is the best grade, because it has the least amount of acidity and highest levels of fatty acids and polyphenols.

Olive oil is one of nature's greatest gifts for preserving your health, beauty, and longevity. When you are buying olive oil, go for the best— extra virgin, cold-pressed olive oil. Not only will you enjoy its richness in your diet but also you will soon see and feel the inestimable benefits in your face and body.

Dairy Products

Milk and dairy products can be an excellent source of protein, calcium, and vitamin D. Look for those that do not contain BGH (bovine growth hormone). I always recommend eating as much organic food as possible, and dairy products are no exception. Of all dairy products, plain yogurt is the best choice as it contains important bacteria for intestinal health and the lactose has been broken down by enzymes making it more easily digestible than milk. Use solid cheeses like Swiss or Cheddar sparingly, as they are calorie dense. Feta cheese is a better choice (once again, the Greeks know best!) and can be crumbled into salads to add flavor. Italian grating cheeses, such as Romano and Parmesan, can also be used to add flavor to salads and other foods. Stay away from those triple crèmes, which are extremely high in fat. I suggest that my adult patients limit their milk intake as they may have lactose intolerance and/or allergies.

The Proinflammatory Vices

By now, we can recite the negative effects of tobacco on the body. We know about the increased risk of lung, mouth, and throat cancer from cigarettes, cigars, and pipes. The effects of smoking in terms of the inflammation–aging-disease connection are significant. When we inhale just one puff of cigarette smoke, more than a trillion free radicals are produced in our lungs, which then trigger an inflammatory response that circulates throughout the body. When cigarette smoke is inhaled, the result is the activation of white blood cells that line our arteries, causing an inflammatory response, predisposing us to heart disease. In addition, there is a tremendous inflammatory response in all the organs of the body. If you are interested in retaining your youth, you must completely avoid smoking. If you currently smoke, it is critical that you stop now.

Alcohol ingestion is another proinflammatory vice. Having a glass of wine with your meal is not a problem, because wine can provide some important antioxidants called polyphenols that do help protect the body. I suggest drinking a glass of wine with your meal, rather than before, to avoid a rapid rise in blood sugar and the ensuing burst of inflammation throughout the body.

Drinking hard liquor causes inflammatory problems in the body. Alcohol is detoxified by the liver. The alcohol content of hard liquor is very high. The metabolites of alcohol are molecules called aldehydes. Aldehydes cause damage to the cell plasma membrane as well as to various portions of the interior of the cell, causing an inflammatory reaction along with this destruction. In summary, wine is fine, but forget the martini.

Take Me to the Water

The fountain of youth did not spew forth diet soda or orange juice—it's always been good old H_2O. If I could teach my patients and students three things that would keep them forever young, they would be 1. drink water; 2. drink water, and 3. drink more water. If you do not drink water, your organs and cells cannot function. How can your skin be soft and plumped up if you refuse the elixir of life? Women and bodybuilders, you will not become bloated if you drink water. In fact, if you don't drink water, you cannot metabolize fat, nor can your body flush wastes from its cells. A dehydrated body provokes the development of aging, inflammatory compounds. In addition, mild dehydration will cause a 3 percent drop in baseline metabolism, resulting in the gain of one pound of fat every six months.

Water is a great weapon to put out the inflammation fire that consumes our youth. I drink at least eight to ten glasses of water a day and urge my patients to do the same. Avoid tap water—it may contain compounds like heavy metals that you don't need (and may be bad for you). And, besides, it does not taste particularly good. Treat yourself to delicious-tasting spring water; there are many to choose from. Avoid chlorinated water whenever possible.

The Right Stuff

When Jack returned two months later, I was delighted to learn that his eczema had improved—and so had his mood. After consulting with his psychiatrist, he was able to drop one of his antidepression medications. Within a year of faithfully following the anti-inflammatory diet and supplement program I outlined, Jack had shown great improvement, both mentally and physically. With his brain functioning clearly and his mood stabilized, Jack has returned to the university as a full-time student. He has resumed his bodybuilding and has had no problem maintaining a healthy ratio between body fat and muscle. His psychiatrist has further reduced his medication. Jack is now looking forward to the day, in the not too distant future, when he can stop the medication altogether.

Jack is an almost perfect textbook example of the seriously detrimental effects of low-fat diets, both to our mental and physical health. As important as the latest medical breakthroughs are to me as a researcher, I consider cases that can be treated with diet and supplements as my greatest, most rewarding successes. Once I can teach my patients how the body works and what it needs to function optimally, they can take charge of their own health, happiness, and longevity.

Now that you understand how the Perricone Wrinkle-Free Diet promotes optimal health, it's time to move on to learning all about the right balance of supplements to maximize the effects of your new lifestyle.

4

Anti-inflammatory Supplements for Smooth and Radiant Skin

An important part of Megan's transformation was rebuilding and rejuvenating her entire body from the inside out. State-of-the-art nutritional supplements tailored to her needs were a key component of the overall plan. Luckily, nutritional supplements have come a long way from the minimal one-size-fits-all one-a-day multivitamins of past generations. Today we have highly targeted antioxidants, amino acids, vitamins, and minerals that can do everything from sharpening brain power, repairing cells, and burning fat to increasing muscle tone, restoring memory, and heightening libido. Many of these superantioxidants penetrate right into the cell where they combat free radicals and decrease inflammation. Because of this, we can honestly state that the right supplements can keep us biologically much younger than our chronological years. In my research I've worked with the world's best nutrient formulators to devise a comprehensive supplement program that restores skin to youthful radiance, improves cognitive function and cellular renewal, and helps reduce body fat. The Perricone Wrinkle-Free Diet, used in conjunction with the supplements you will learn about in this chapter, results in a potent, anti-aging, skin-rejuvenating formula.

Although essential fatty acids (EFAs) were discussed at length in the previous chapter, they are so crucial to skin health that they merit further mention. EFAs were once known as "vitamin F," because they are considered essential to controlling the body oils, the fats, and lipids that keep skin soft, smooth, and youthful—and, like vitamins, they must be obtained from foods or supplements. And, remember, you can't get "vitamin F" from a fat-free diet. In fact, EFA deficiencies are a major concern with extreme low-fat diets.

Making nutrient-deficient food choices results in more than just fatigue and depression; poor diet is reflected in your skin as pallor, puffiness, and dark under-eye circles. Your skin is composed of rapidly dividing cells, making it especially sensitive to nutrient status. Good health and beautiful skin go hand in hand, and the targeted supplementation can help you achieve and maintain both.

On the Perricone Wrinkle-Free supplement program, you may be taking more pills than you are accustomed to. To ensure that you maintain therapeutic levels in your blood, vitamins should be taken more than once a day. One simple way to keep track is to use an inexpensive weekly pill sorter, available at your pharmacy. If I am having a busy day or eating out, I take the pills I need, sorted by dose into individual miniature manila envelopes (these can be found in any office supply store). To make it even easier, I have developed a complete supplement program in packets that can be taken twice a day and contain all the recommended nutrients for the Perricone Wrinkle-Free Program. Supplementation should be as routine and consistent as brushing your teeth. Make taking these pills a habit—something you do automatically, without a second thought. If you take the vitamins in the doses I recommend each day, you will see great improvements in your skin and energy level.

The Brain-Beauty Connection

What is the exact connection between our brains and our skin? And why is it that so many nutrients that are key to proper brain function, good mental health, and well-being are the same nutrients that give us healthy, glowing skin? As a research scien-

continued on next page

tist and a dermatologist, I have observed that if something has a positive effect on the central nervous system—whether it is a nutrient, herb, or any pharmacological agent—it seems also to have a positive effect on the skin.

It all starts in the womb. When a fetus develops, all of its tissue is derived from three distinct layers of cells. The same layer of tissue from which the brain is derived is also the source of the skin. Consequently, there is a strong connection between the two structures.

This chapter is designed for quick and easy reference for all the nutrients we need, including:

- A list of the features and benefits of that nutrient
- The symptoms and effects of a deficiency in that nutrient
- The best noninflammatory food sources
- The reference daily intake (RDI). In most cases, the RDI doses are identical to the U.S. RDA doses—we use them here since federal law requires manufacturers to express the amount of nutrient in terms of the percent of the RDI. The RDIs are the minimum doses needed to prevent nutrient-deficiency symptoms. I generally recommend doses of vitamins and minerals somewhat higher than the RDI levels.
- The no observed adverse effects level (NOAEL) is the maximum daily dose that does not produce adverse effects, according to the Council for Responsible Nutrition. Certain nutrients are safe, and more supportive of optimal health, at even higher doses (for example, high-dose niacin for improving blood cholesterol levels)—levels that may, in some circumstances, produce noninjurious adverse effects. The NOAEL doses are the maximums I would ever recommend. Pregnant or lactating women should not exceed the RDI, except under a doctor's direction.
- The Wrinkle-Free Recommendation is the daily dose the average healthy adult needs to take to receive the maximum health and

cosmetic benefits each supplement can provide. Check with your physician to be sure that these doses are appropriate for your individual health status—and will not interact negatively with any medications you take.

At the end of the chapter, there is a schedule of supplements for you to take daily on the 28-Day Wrinkle-Free Program and for the rest of your life. In the Resources appendix, you will find a list of companies from which you can order the vitamins for the program. It is impractical to replicate the exact balance found in my Skin and Total Body Nutritional Supplements, but the vitamins recommended on this schedule will work to fight inflammation and to make your skin glow with health.

Alpha Lipoic Acid: The Universal and Metabolic Antioxidant

Before covering the ABCs of nutritional supplements, I want to tell you about a natural substance found in our bodies known as alpha lipoic acid—one of the most powerful antiaging, antioxidant, anti-inflammatories available.

FEATURES AND BENEFITS
- Assists energy production in the cell
- Fat and water soluble; works in both the fatty cell plasma membrane and the aqueous interior of the cell
- Helps regenerate vitamin C and E
- Protects DNA (the cells' genetic instructions)
- Protects the mitochondria (the energy-producing portion of cell)
- Inhibits the activation of transcription factor NF-kB, reducing cellular inflammation
- Controls AP-1, helps to remodel collagen
- Protects the skin from free radical initiation of inflammation including sun exposure
- Increases cellular energy and vitality

- Inhibits glycosylation (the abnormal attachment of sugar to protein), which results in cross-linking of collagen making it stiff and inflexible
- Acts synergistically with all antioxidant systems
- Protects and elevates glutathione, an antioxidant inside the cells
- Acts as a powerful anti-inflammatory agent
- Accelerates the removal of glucose from the bloodstream
- Improves insulin function
- Decreases insulin resistance
- Inhibits replication of HIV in the test tube

INTAKE REQUIREMENTS AND SUPPLEMENT RECOMMENDATIONS
- RDA: none established
- Wrinkle-Free Recommendation: 200 mg, divided in two doses: 100 mg at breakfast and 100 mg at lunch

Alpha lipoic acid is called the "universal antioxidant" because it is both fat and water soluble. Further, it is four hundred times stronger than vitamins E and C combined (both of which are renowned for their antioxidant properties). Alpha lipoic acid readily penetrates the cell plasma membrane and the plasma membranes that surround such key parts of the cell as the mitochondria and the nucleus. Since alpha lipoic acid is also water soluble, it can get into the cytosol. By penetrating the inside and the outside of the cell, alpha lipoic acid brings protection wherever it is needed.

The body contains small amounts of alpha lipoic acid inside the mitochondria. It exists as part of an energy-producing enzyme system called the pyruvate dehydrogenase complex. This enzyme system helps convert food to energy; however it is important to note that alpha lipoic acid remains locked within this system and does not float freely in the cell.

However, if you take alpha lipoic acid as a supplement in capsule form, or apply it topically as a lotion, it performs as an antioxidant as well as an aid to cellular metabolism. Alpha lipoic acid boosts energy production in your cells, just as it helps the mitochondria change food to energy. As you know the higher the energy level in the cell, the more youthful

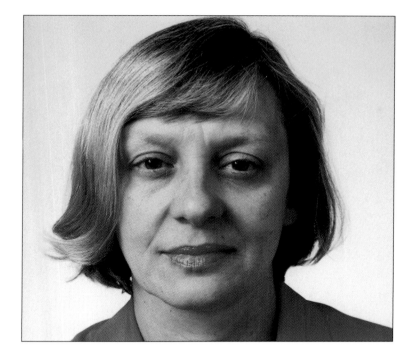

THREE-DAY NUTRITIONAL FACE-LIFT

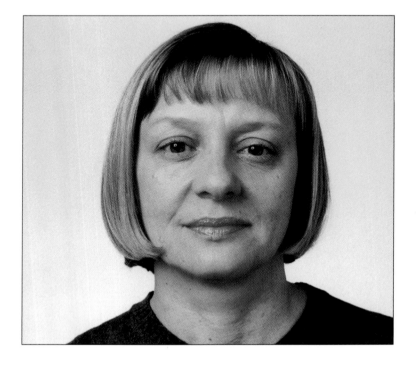

HAIRCUT ASIDE, look at the difference in this woman's face in just three days. The lines between her eyes are not as deep, the puffiness has been reduced. Her overall skin tone is more refined and radiant. Her jawline is firmer.

THREE-DAY NUTRITIONAL FACE-LIFT

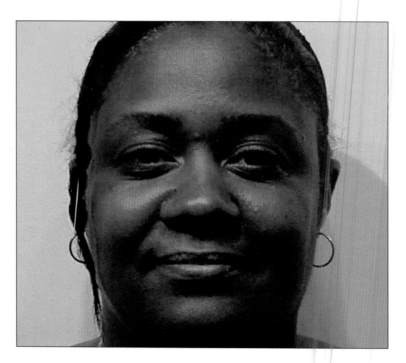

LOOK AT WHAT JUST three days can do. This woman's skin tone has become considerably more even, her pores smaller. The puffiness above her eyes has been reduced. Her blemishes—particularly the one on the bridge of her nose—have vanished. Her nasolabial folds are no longer as deep.

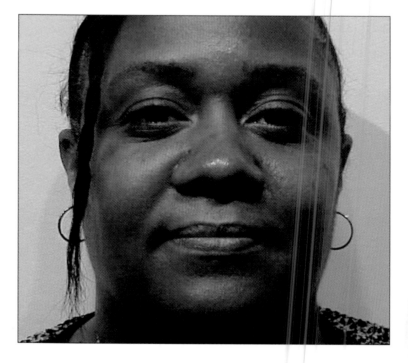

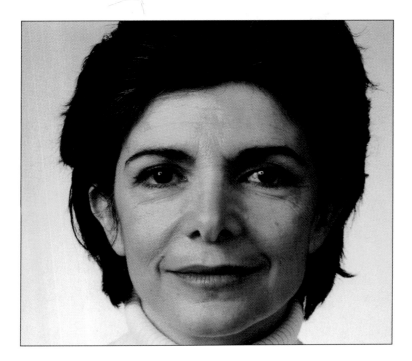

THREE-DAY NUTRITIONAL FACE-LIFT

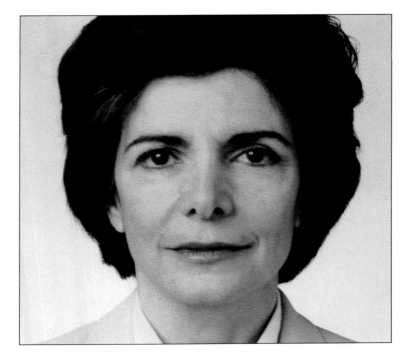

THIS WOMAN'S SKIN is so much smoother. The lines on her forehead, the lines between her eyebrows, and the bags under her eyes have diminished. Her skin tone is more even. The nasolabial folds have improved, particularly on the left side of her face.

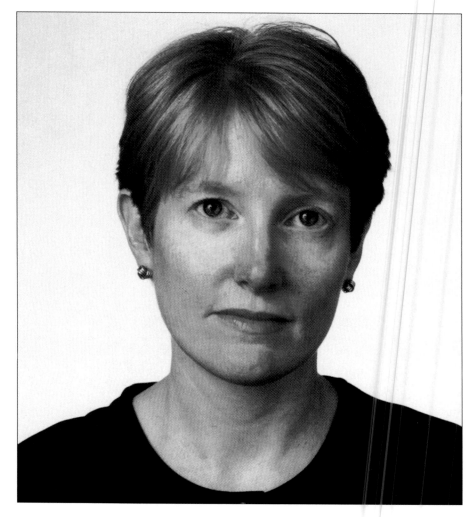

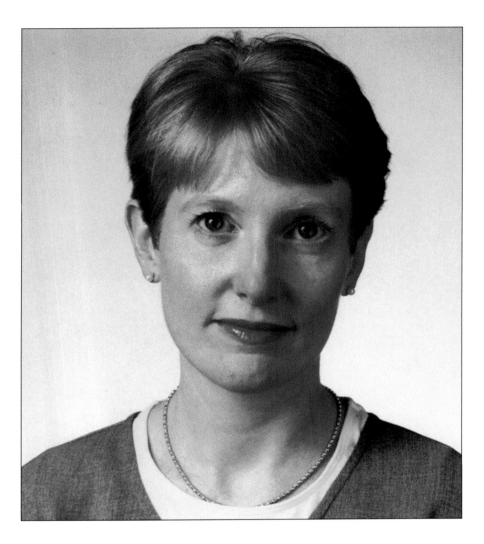

THE IMPROVEMENT IN THIS WOMAN'S JAWLINE AND NECK AFTER TWENTY-EIGHT days is remarkable. The puffiness around her eyes has been reduced and her crow's-feet are much less deep. Her skin is glowing rather than ruddy as in the before shot.

28-DAY WRINKLE-FREE PROGRAM

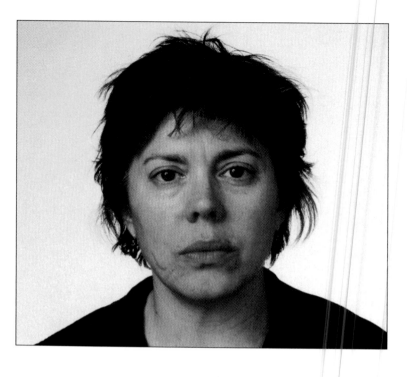

THIS WOMAN'S SKIN tone has evened out quite well. The hooded look of her upper eyelids is reduced and the brow is lifted. Her neck and jawline are much better defined. Her skin looks much younger.

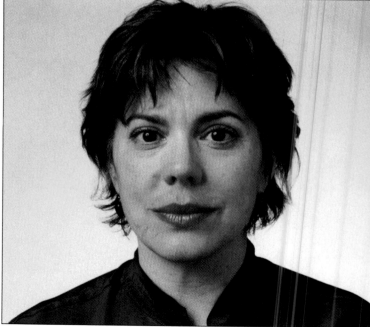

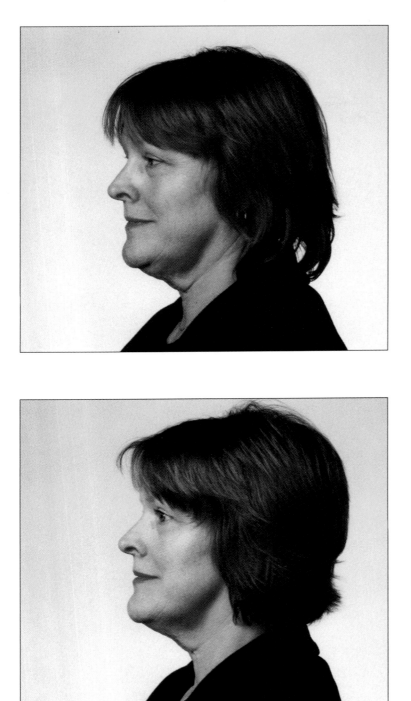

THIS WOMAN'S SKIN now radiates health. The contours of her face have improved significantly. Her neck is firmer as well. Weight loss has also improved facial contours.

28-DAY WRINKLE-FREE PROGRAM

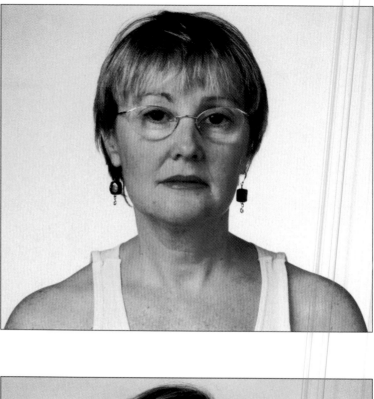

LOOK AT HOW THE redness of this woman's skin has diminished. She has better jawline definition and her nasolabial folds are not as deep.

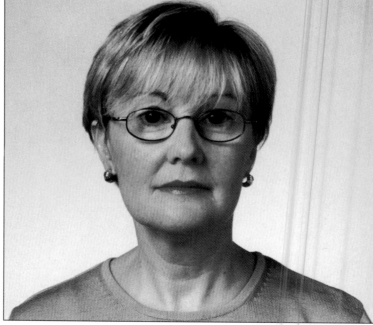

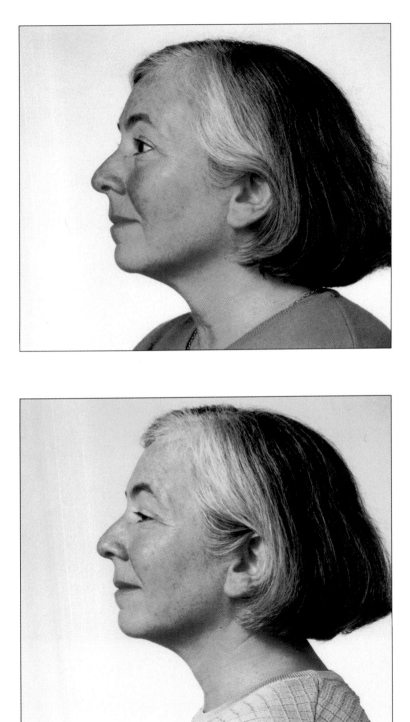

SKIN TONE IS THE
great improvement
here. The redness
is gone, and her
skin seems to glow.
Her jawline is
more defined.

28-DAY
WRINKLE-FREE
PROGRAM

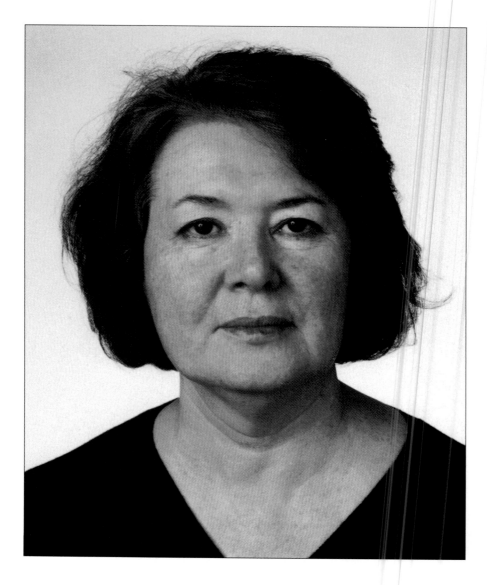

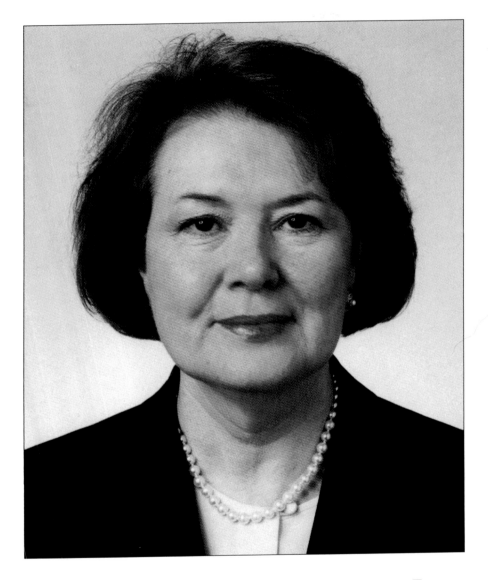

WHAT AN IMPROVEMENT IN CONTOURS THIS WOMAN'S FACE SHOWS. THERE IS an all-over lift to her face. Her very fair, sensitive skin went from being red and burned looking to rosy and glowing.

28-DAY WRINKLE-FREE PROGRAM

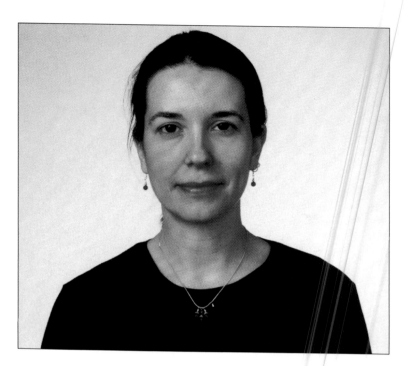

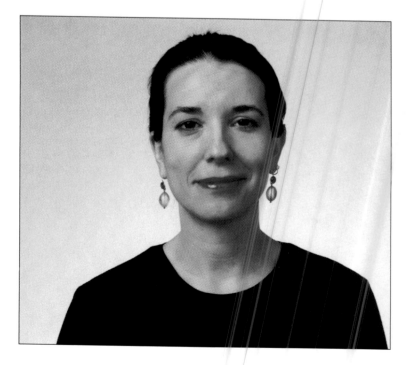

FROM LOOKING tired to radiant, this woman's skin tone has evened out, and she seems to glow from within. Her blemishes have subsided.

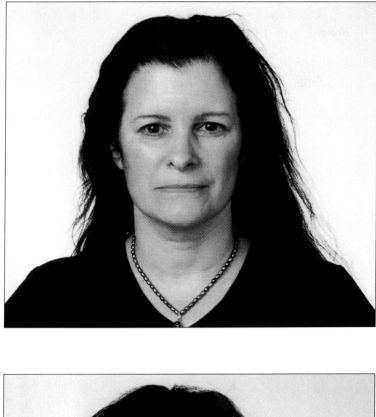

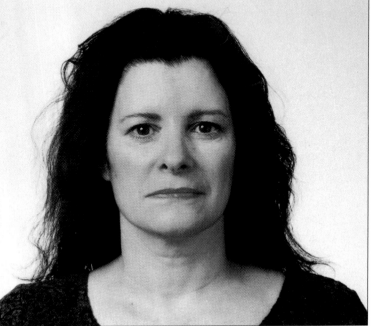

THIS WOMAN'S brows have lifted and her eyes appear wider. The bags under her eyes have been reduced. Her skin has a richer tone, and her neck is improved.

28-DAY
WRINKLE-FREE
PROGRAM

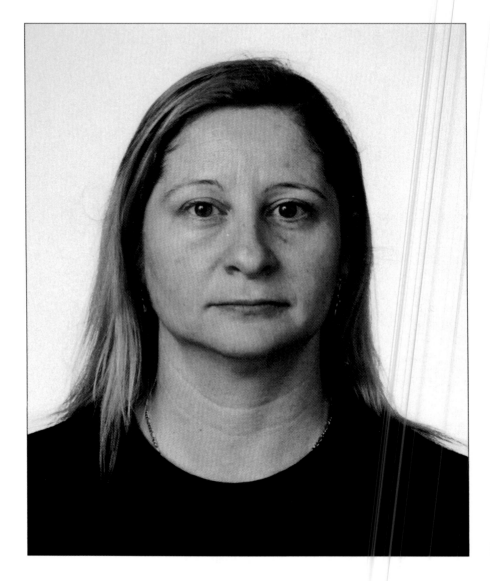

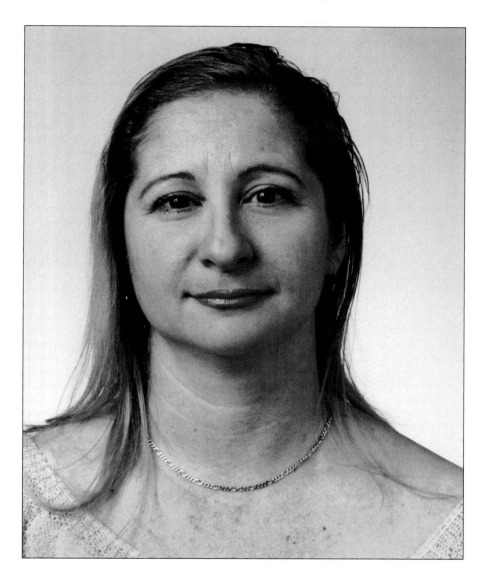

THIS WOMAN'S ENTIRE FACE HAS BEEN LIFTED. HER SKIN IS MORE REFINED, HER EYES appear larger. Her skin has lost its dullness and is now vibrant.

28-DAY WRINKLE-FREE PROGRAM

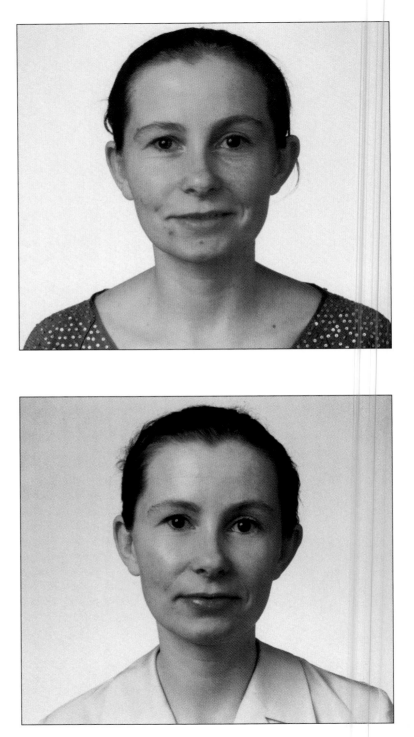

THIS WOMAN'S FACIAL blemishes are resolved. There is a marked increase in radiance. Her jawline looks firmer.

SIXTEEN WEEKS
Johnson & Johnson Clinical Trial of DMAE

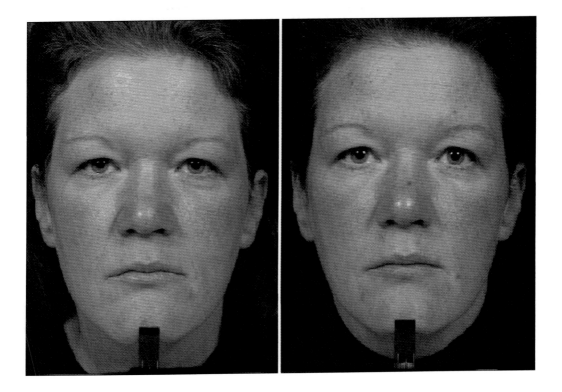

NOTICE THE DIFFERENCE IN THE FOREHEAD WRINKLES OF THIS SUBJECT. THE AFTER PHOTO shows fewer, more superficial lines. The after photo even shows a lift in those lines and the brows are higher and the upper-eye puffiness is reduced, resulting in bigger eyes. The under-eye area is smoother, its skin looks thicker. The line on the bridge of the nose has diminished. The nasolabial folds do not extend as far. The face looks less droopy, more contoured overall. The skin above the lips is smoother. The line beneath the lower lip is no longer there. Her skin looks firmer and more vibrant.

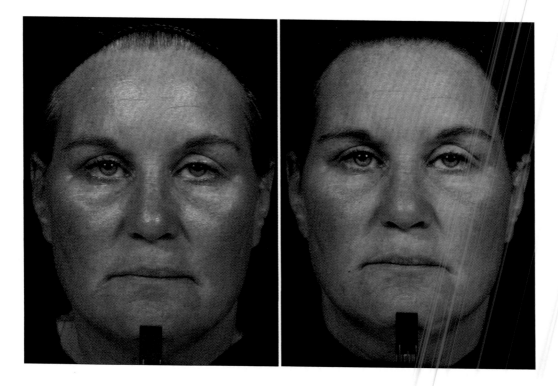

THIS SUBJECT'S FACIAL RUDDINESS HAS DISAPPEARED, AN OBVIOUS SIGN OF A REDUCTION in inflammation. Her pores have shrunk, resulting in a more refined look. The skin under her eyes has thickened and the bags are reduced. The upper eyelid puffiness has gone down, resulting in higher brows, particularly on the right side of the after photo. The contours of the cheeks have improved and her jaw is firmer. Her nasolabial folds are not as deep. Her upper lip is much smoother. Even the lines at the sides of her mouth have diminished. The overall tone of her skin is smoother.

SIXTEEN WEEKS

Johnson & Johnson Clinical Trial of DMAE

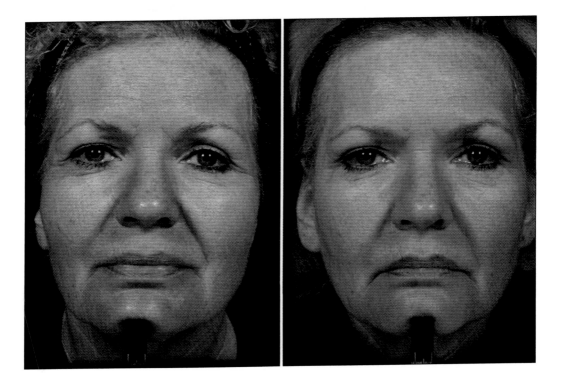

LOOK AT THE BIG DIFFERENCE IN THIS SUBJECT'S EYES. HER CROW'S-FEET AND UNDER-EYE wrinkles have been significantly reduced. Her brows are higher. The puffiness has abated, making her eyes look bigger and less droopy. The forehead wrinkles have vanished. Her jaw is sharper, better defined as is her nose. Her pores are smaller. Unfortunately, the expression of her mouth is different, so it is difficult to fully judge improvement.

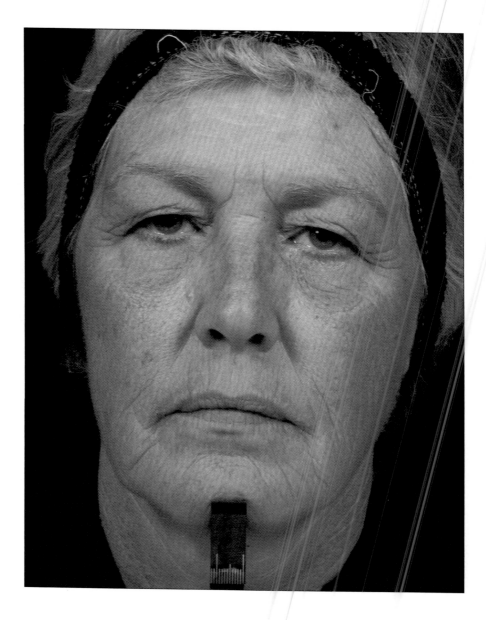

NOTICE THE SIGNIFICANT REDUCTION IN THE CROW'S-FEET, WRINKLES BETWEEN the eyes and around the entire eye area, the nasolabial folds, the wrinkles on the upper lip, the corners of the mouth, and the neck. Her face is so much smoother. The skin tone has improved a good deal. Her face is no longer saggy. If you look at the far right of the after photo, you can see that her face is plumped up even more. Her pores are reduced. The redness is gone and an even color has returned.

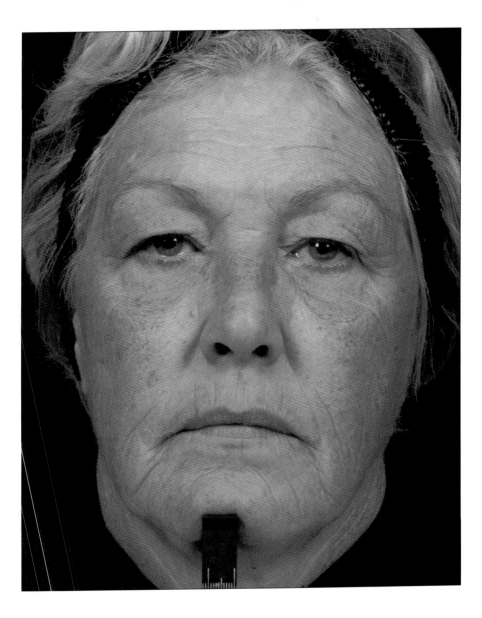

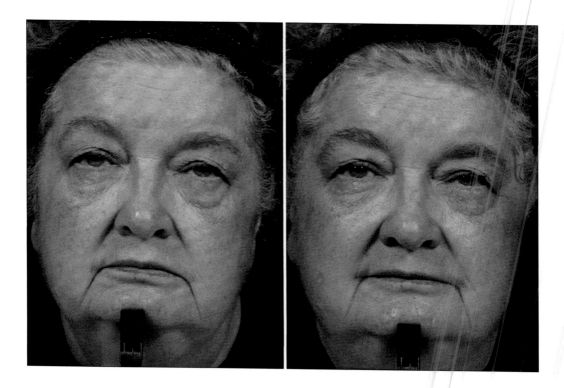

THE CREPEY QUALITY OF THIS SUBJECT'S SKIN HAS CHANGED DRAMATICALLY. HER SKIN HAS become more vibrant, losing its dullness and pallor. There has been an all-over lift to the face. The puffiness around her eyes has been reduced, decreasing their hooded appearance.

FIFTY-TWO WEEKS

Johnson & Johnson Clinical Trial of DMAE

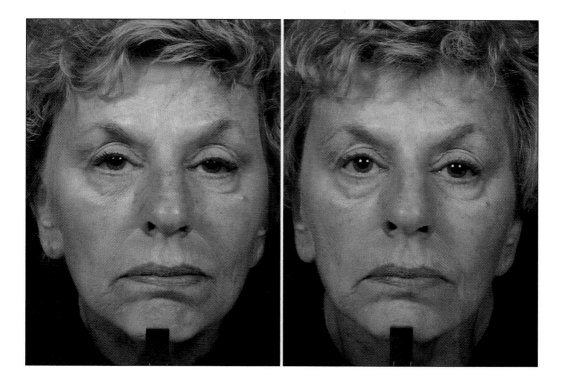

THE OVERALL LIFT OF THIS WOMAN'S FACE IS REMARKABLE. HER EYES ARE LESS HOODED. The fine wrinkles under her eyes are gone. Her nasolabial folds have receded. Her pores are smaller, and the overall look of her skin is more refined.

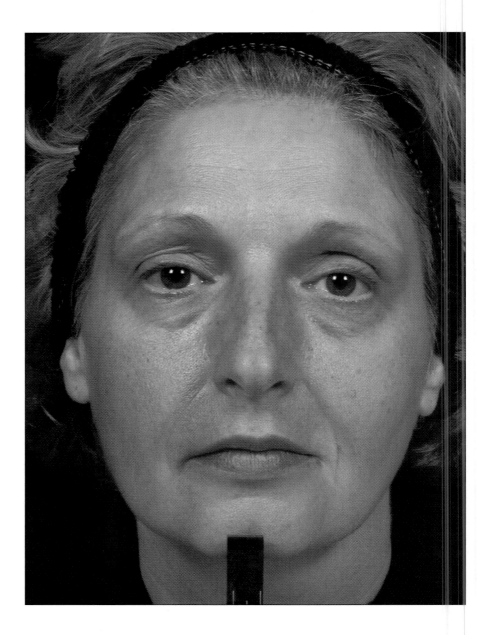

THE MOST STRIKING CHANGE IN THIS WOMAN'S FACE IS THAT IT IS PLUMPED UP. Her fine lines have vanished. Her skin tone is smoother and more even and her pores appear smaller and more refined. The wrinkles around her eyes have diminished.

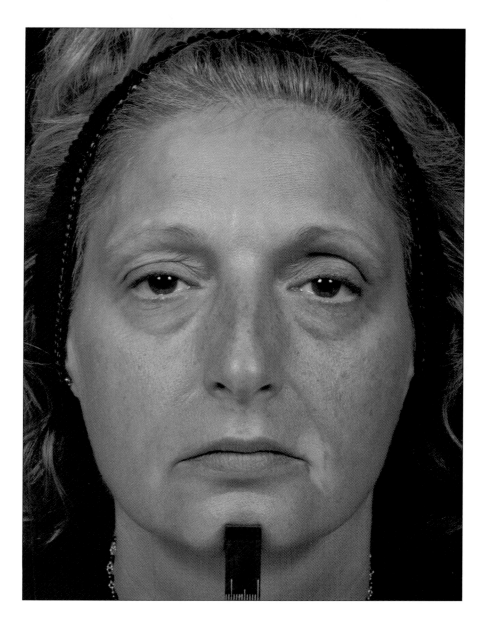

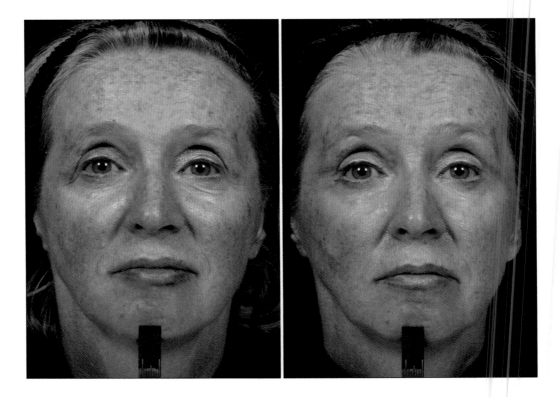

THE CONTOURS OF THIS WOMAN'S FACE HAVE IMPROVED GREATLY, AND HER FACE IS LIFTED. The redness has subsided. Her under-eye wrinkles have diminished. Her crow's-feet have vanished. Weight loss is evident in the increased jawline definition.

FIFTY-TWO WEEKS
Johnson & Johnson Clinical Trial of DMAE

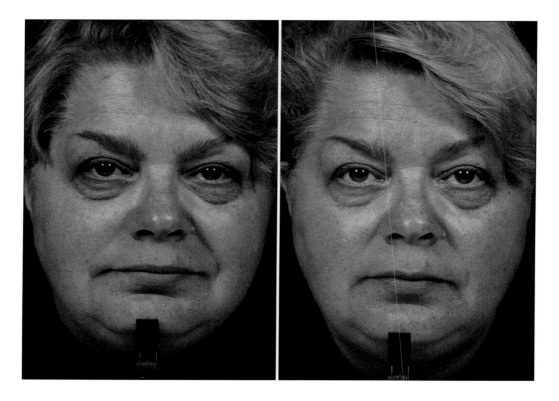

THE OVERALL REFINEMENT VISIBLE IN THIS WOMAN'S FACE IS STRIKING. HER PORES ARE reduced. Her facial features are more refined. Her skin tone is more even. The wrinkles in her forehead are diminished. The neck and chin reflect overall weight loss.

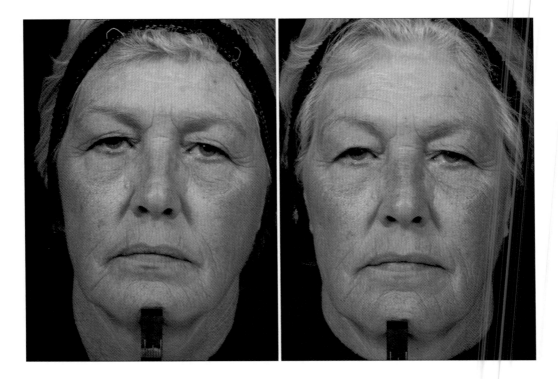

A SIGNIFICANT WEIGHT LOSS IS EVIDENT IN THIS WOMAN'S FACE. THE PUFFINESS AROUND her eyes has been reduced as have the bags under her eyes, the result of a decrease in inflammation. The fine lines around her eyes are gone. Her nasolabial folds have shortened. Her skin tone has improved because the redness is gone. Increased tone has lifted the forehead.

too high in sodium. Instead, use only fresh garlic, onions, and scallions for seasoning. Others, such as chili mix, are high in sugar and salt. Health food stores sell herbs and spices in bulk, allowing you to purchase them in small quantities to ensure freshness. Grocery stores now sell a wide variety of fresh herbs that will add wonderful flavor to your meals.

Recommended herbs
- Basil
- Bay leaf
- Dill
- Mint
- Oregano
- Rosemary
- Thyme

Recommended spices
- Cinnamon
- Coriander
- Cumin
- Ginger (fresh and ground)
- Paprika
- Red pepper flakes (dried)
- Turmeric

Phase II Preparation: The Supplements

Check the expiration dates on all your vitamins and throw out all those that have expired. In addition, check the dosages to make certain they fit within my recommendations. Make sure you have adequate supplies of the supplements recommended on the Wrinkle-Free Program on page 104 in Chapter Four.

Follow the daily supplement schedule and sort your vitamins a week at a time. As I mentioned earlier, you can use a weekly pill sorter or small brown envelopes marked "breakfast," "lunch," and "bedtime," or the preprepared vitamin packets recommended in Appendix B. A little simple preparation will help keep supplements a part of your daily routine—and keep your body supplied with essential nutrients.

Always take your pills with a full glass of water (at least eight ounces). A supplement icon

appears in the daily plan whenever supplements are scheduled to be taken.

Phase III Preparation: The Topicals

Rid your bathroom shelves and bureau top of harsh facial cleansers, scrubs, and astringents and old creams and expired sunscreen.

Go to the drugstore, department store, a specialty cosmetic store, or online to order the skin care products you need to fight inflammation and restore your skin's youthful glow.

Make choices appropriate for your skin color; select from the products recommended on the chart on page 139. The daily plans will have an icon to remind you to follow the program for skin care. It looks like this:

Phase IV Preparation: Workout Gear

Make sure you have comfortable, loose-fitting clothes, good running shoes, and cushioned socks for your workouts. You will also need dumbbells. Start with two-pound weights if you have never done weight training. If you have, you know your weight level. You'll also need two-pound ankle weights. An exercise mat is optional, but it's a good idea to have one.

Set aside thirty minutes each day at a time that is most convenient

you remain. The importance of alpha lipoic acid—the metabolic antioxidant—is hard to overstate.

I have to get technical to explain another important function of alpha lipoic acid. It inhibits the action of transcription factor NF-kB, which you learned about in the previous chapter. Alpha lipoic acid can "scoop up" free radicals before they attack the polyunsaturated fats in the cell plasma membrane, thus preventing the formation of dangerous oxidized fats called lipid peroxides. As you remember, these toxic lipids trigger damage to DNA and the activation of NF-kB.

Under normal conditions, NF-kB is a harmless protein molecule that remains inert thanks to an inhibitor attachment. But when a cell is in a state of oxidative stress, the inhibitor portion detaches, allowing NF-kB to migrate to the nucleus. There, NF-kB turns on transcription (it allows DNA to give instructions to the cell) causing production of proinflammatory chemicals called cytokines (such as tumor necrosis factor alpha and interleukins).

The good news is that alpha lipoic acid inhibits the activation of NF-kB better than any other antioxidant. It blocks the production of enzymes that damage the collagen fibers, preserving a smooth skin surface. It is equally effective in preventing glycation, the harmful effects of sugar molecules on collagen fibers.

Remember AP-1 from the previous chapter? Alpha lipoic acid has a tremendous effect on that transcription factor, too. When AP-1 is turned on by oxidative stress created by sunlight, it actually digests your collagen, causing microscars. But when AP-1 is activated by alpha lipoic acid, it turns on the production of collagen-digesting enzymes that digest *damaged* rather than healthy collagen. That process helps to remodel scar tissue.

Knowledge is power, and I believe it is important for you to have a good, basic understanding of these biochemical and biological "miracles," so you will be inspired to stay on the Wrinkle-Free Program. If I simply say, "eat this" or "take that," you might follow the plan for a while—until the day you're tempted by a fast food "fix" or a piece of chocolate cake. So use the information in this book to paint a vivid mental picture of how diet affects your overall health and energy. Once you really "get" that unavoidable reality, you can transform the way you look and the rate at which you age for the rest of your life.

Vitamins: Starting with the ABCs

Vitamins are either fat soluble or water soluble. Vitamins A, D, E, and K are fat soluble. They are stored in the liver and used up by the body very slowly. A buildup of these fat-soluble vitamins can be toxic. The B-complex vitamins and vitamin C are water soluble. The body uses these vitamins very quickly and excess amounts are eliminated in the urine. Vitamin A, the B-complex vitamins, and vitamin C are the foundation of my nutritional antiaging regimen.

Vitamin A

FEATURES AND BENEFITS
- Fat soluble
- Essential for growth
- Aids bone development
- Strengthens immune system
- Improves night vision
- Helps reproduction
- Promotes wound healing
- Encourages healthy skin

SYMPTOMS AND EFFECTS OF A VITAMIN A DEFICIENCY
- Disorder of the eyes and epithelial tissues (the skin and mucous membranes lining the internal body surfaces)
- Rough, dry skin

NONINFLAMMATORY FOOD SOURCES
- Broccoli
- Cantaloupe
- Cod

- Halibut
- Kale
- Red bell peppers
- Spinach
- Watercress

INTAKE REQUIREMENTS AND SUPPLEMENT RECOMMENDATIONS

- RDI: 5,000 IU
- No observed adverse effects level: 10,000 IU
- Wrinkle-Free recommendation: 5,000 to 10,000 IU from carotenoid sources

Vitamin A is part of a group of compounds called retinoids. It is found in animal products like liver, dairy products, eggs, and fish liver oil; it is also found in dark-red, green, and yellow vegetables. Vitamin A is best absorbed in the presence of some dietary fat and with sufficient zinc, vitamin E, and protein in the body. As with all fat-soluble vitamins, excessive intake of vitamin A is toxic—unless you take it in the form of carotenes that the body converts to vitamin A on an as-needed basis.

Vitamin A helps cells reproduce normally, in a process known as differentiation. Cells that have not properly differentiated are more likely to undergo precancerous changes. Vitamin A is important for the health and integrity of the cell plasma membrane. As a fat-soluble antioxidant, it can get into the cell, provide protection, neutralize free radicals, and prevent oxidative stress.

A half-cup serving of broccoli, spinach, or cantaloupe contains enough vitamin A (in its precursor form, carotene) to meet the RDA for this nutrient. For antioxidant benefits, I recommend between 5,000 and 10,000 IU of vitamin A each day. Bear in mind that the liver stores vitamin A—and a buildup can be toxic. To avoid problems, do not exceed dosage recommendations for this and other fat-soluble vitamins. It is also important to note that many foods that are high in vitamin A (as carotenes) can cause an inflammatory response as a result of their high sugar content. These include sweet potatoes, carrots, and yams, which I recommend you avoid.

The most popular prescription for acne and aging skin is topical Retin-A (tretinoin), an acid form of vitamin A. Retinol, the alcohol form of vitamin A, is used in cosmetics because it is converted in the skin into small amounts of tretinoin.

Vitamin B Complex

FEATURES AND BENEFITS

- Increased health of skin, hair, and nails
- Strengthens bones and muscle
- Improves energy production
- Helps metabolic function
- Aids protein digestion
- Promotes nervous system health
- Fortifies mucosal membranes
- Stimulates healthy intestinal and bowel function
- Prevents moodiness, restlessness, irritability, insomnia, and fatigue
- Improves liver health
- Reinforces proper brain cell function
- Prevents skin disorders
- Relieves PMS

SYMPTOMS AND EFFECTS OF A VITAMIN B-COMPLEX DEFICIENCY

- Many skin disorders
- Nervousness
- Depression
- Lethargy
- Forgetfulness
- Insomnia

There are eight B vitamins in the Wrinkle-Free supplement program:

- Vitamin B_1 (thiamin)
- Vitamin B_2 (riboflavin)

- Vitamin B_3 (niacin)
- Vitamin B_5 (pantothenic acid)
- Vitamin B_6 (pyridoxine)
- Vitamin B_{12} (cyanocobalamin)
- Folic Acid (folate)
- Biotin

Most of the B vitamins are recognized as coenzymes that, taken together, work synergistically to perform essential biological processes—especially those affecting the nerves, brain, and skin.

This group of vitamins is water soluble, which means that they are not stored in the body and must be replenished each day. Let's take a closer look at each of the B vitamins.

Vitamin B_1 (Thiamin)

FEATURES AND BENEFITS

- Stimulates conversion of carbohydrates and glucose into energy
- Helps metabolism of proteins and fats
- Promotes healthy growth during childhood and adolescence
- Aids digestion
- Improves mental attitude
- Promotes normal function of the nervous system, muscles, and heart

SYMPTOMS AND EFFECTS OF A VITAMIN B_1 DEFICIENCY

- Problems with gastrointestinal, cardiovascular, and peripheral nervous systems
- Depression
- Irritability
- Attention deficit
- Muscular weakness

NONINFLAMMATORY FOOD SOURCES

- Chickpeas
- Pinto beans
- Raw nuts

- Salmon
- Soybeans

INTAKE REQUIREMENTS AND SUPPLEMENT RECOMMENDATIONS
- RDI: 1.5 mg
- No observed adverse effects level: 50 mg
- Wrinkle-Free recommendation: 10 to 50 mg

Vitamin B_2 (Riboflavin)

FEATURES AND BENEFITS
- Essential for normal cell growth
- Helps metabolize carbohydrates, fats, and proteins
- Promotes healthy skin, hair, and nails

SYMPTOMS AND EFFECTS OF A VITAMIN B_2 DEFICIENCY
- Sores and cracks at the corners of the mouth
- Inflammation of the tongue and skin

NONINFLAMMATORY FOOD SOURCES
- Almonds
- Low-fat cottage cheese
- Low-fat milk
- Plain yogurt
- Walnuts

INTAKE REQUIREMENTS AND SUPPLEMENT RECOMMENDATIONS
- RDI: 1.7 mg
- No observed adverse effects level: 200 mg
- Wrinkle-Free recommendation: 10 to 100 mg

Vitamin B_3 (Niacin)

FEATURES AND BENEFITS
- Aids cellular and lipid metabolism
- Maintains healthy skin
- Helps synthesize hormones

- Supports gastrointestinal and nervous system health
- Protects against carcinogens, preventing certain types of cancer
- Reduces cholesterol and triglyceride levels
- Treats and prevents circulatory problems
- Maintains mental stability

SYMPTOMS AND EFFECTS OF A VITAMIN B_3 DEFICIENCY
- Dermatitis
- Diarrhea
- Dementia
- Eye redness
- Loss of appetite
- Anxiety or nervousness

NONINFLAMMATORY FOOD SOURCES
- Almonds
- Hazelnuts
- Plain yogurt
- Sunflower seeds

INTAKE REQUIREMENTS AND SUPPLEMENT RECOMMENDATIONS
- RDI: 20 mg
- No observed adverse effects level: 500 mg (Note: Doses of 1,000 to 4,000 mg a day are used for cholesterol control, and, while generally safe, may produce side effects such as hot flushes, nausea, and heartburn. Never take more than 500 mg a day of niacin without medical supervision.)
- Wrinkle-Free recommendation: 20 to 100 mg

Vitamin B_5 (Pantothenic Acid)
FEATURES AND BENEFITS
- Promotes Krebs cycle of energy production (takes place in the mitochondria)
- Helps production of adrenal hormones
- Reduces cholesterol and triglyceride levels

- Plays a role in metabolism of fats, carbohydrates, and proteins
- Helps fight infection
- Increases physical endurance
- Improves body's ability to heal
- Helps create antibodies
- Improves digestion
- Aids nervous system operation, adrenal gland function, glandular balance

SYMPTOMS AND EFFECTS OF A VITAMIN B$_5$ DEFICIENCY
- Fatigue
- Muscle cramps
- Stomach pain
- Vomiting

NONINFLAMMATORY FOOD SOURCES
- Almonds
- Black beans
- Chickpeas
- Lentils

INTAKE REQUIREMENTS AND SUPPLEMENT RECOMMENDATIONS
- RDI: 10 mg
- No observed adverse effects level: 1,000 mg
- Wrinkle-Free recommendation: 10 to 250 mg

Vitamin B$_6$ (Pyridoxine)
FEATURES AND BENEFITS
- Required for function of more than sixty enzymes
- Essential for processing amino acids
- Helps in the formation of several neurotransmitters
- Essential for regulation of mental processes that influence mood
- Lowers homocysteine levels—a substance linked to cardiovascular disease, stroke, osteoporosis, and Alzheimer's disease (in combination with folic acid and B$_{12}$)

- Helps synthesize fatty acids
- Helps metabolize cholesterol
- Used to produce neurotransmitters, including serotonin, melatonin, and dopamine
- Crucial for a healthy immune system
- Maintains blood sugar within a normal range

SYMPTOMS AND EFFECTS OF A VITAMIN B_6 DEFICIENCY
- Dermatitis
- Glossitis (sore tongue)
- Depression
- Confusion
- Convulsions

NONINFLAMMATORY FOOD SOURCES
- Eggs
- Lentils
- Pinto beans
- Salmon

INTAKE REQUIREMENTS AND SUPPLEMENT RECOMMENDATIONS
- RDI: 2 mg
- No observed adverse effects level: 200 mg
- Wrinkle-Free recommendation: 50 to 100 mg

Vitamin B_{12} (Cyanocobalamin)
FEATURES AND BENEFITS
- Functions in the gastrointestinal tract, the nervous system, and the bone marrow
- Helps maintain healthy nerve cells and red blood cells
- Needed to make DNA
- Lowers homocysteine levels (in combination with folic acid and B_6)

SYMPTOMS AND EFFECTS OF A VITAMIN B_{12} DEFICIENCY

- Pernicious anemia
- Fatigue
- Weakness
- Nausea
- Constipation
- Flatulence
- Loss of appetite
- Weight loss
- Numbness and tingling in the hands and feet
- Deficiency often occurs in vegetarians who eat no animal products

NONINFLAMMATORY FOOD SOURCES

- Eggs
- Halibut
- Plain yogurt
- Salmon

INTAKE REQUIREMENTS AND SUPPLEMENT RECOMMENDATIONS

- RDI: 6 mcg
- No observed adverse effects level: 3,000 mcg
- Wrinkle-Free recommendation: 5 to 100 mcg

Folic Acid (Folate)

FEATURES AND BENEFITS

- Necessary for synthesis of nucleic acids
- Aids in the formation of red blood cells
- Lowers homocysteine levels (in combination with B_{12} and B_6)

SYMPTOMS AND EFFECTS OF A FOLIC ACID DEFICIENCY

- Insufficient and enlarged red blood cells (megaloblastic anemia)
- Gastrointestinal problems
- Sore tongue
- Cracks at corners of mouth

- Diarrhea
- Ulceration of stomach and intestines

NONINFLAMMATORY FOOD SOURCES
- Asparagus
- Avocado
- Beet
- Black beans
- Brussels sprouts
- Cauliflower
- Chicken breast
- Chickpeas
- Dried beans
- Kale
- Kidney beans
- Melon
- Orange
- Parsnips
- Spinach

INTAKE REQUIREMENTS AND SUPPLEMENT RECOMMENDATIONS
- RDI: 400 mcg
- No observed adverse effects level: 1,000 mcg
- Wrinkle-Free recommendation: 400 to 800 mcg

Biotin
FEATURES AND BENEFITS
- Helps metabolism of fats, carbohydrates, and proteins
- Aids in utilization of folic acid, vitamin B_5, and vitamin B_1
- Promotes healthy hair

SYMPTOMS AND EFFECTS OF A BIOTIN DEFICIENCY
- Anorexia
- Nausea
- Vomiting

- Inflammation of the tongue
- Gray pallor
- Depression
- Hair loss
- Dermatitis

INTAKE REQUIREMENTS AND SUPPLEMENT RECOMMENDATIONS
- RDI: 300 mcg (Note: Biotin supplements should be taken when the daily intake of alpha lipoic acid exceeds 100 mg. This is because alpha lipoic acid can compete with biotin and in the long run, interfere with biotin's activities in the body.)
- No observed adverse effects level: 2,500 mcg
- Wrinkle-Free recommendation: 300 mcg

Vitamin C

Vitamin C is another superstar in the pantheon of antioxidant age fighters. There are two basic types of vitamin C, and each makes important contributions.

The form of vitamin C with which people are most familiar is L-ascorbic acid, which is water soluble. As a water-soluble vitamin, L-ascorbic acid protects the cytosol, the watery interior of the cell.

But there is a fat-soluble form of vitamin C called vitamin C ester. (The best known vitamin C ester—and the ester I prescribe for topical use—is ascorbyl palmitate.) Vitamin C ester protects the fatty portions of the cell that are not protected by L-ascorbic acid.

Vitamin C: One Kind for Your Inside, Another for Your Outside

There is much confusion about a fat-soluble form of vitamin C called vitamin C ester. An ester is a chemical compound that combines an acid and an alcohol. Ascorbyl palmitate—the best known ester of vitamin C—is made by adding a fatty acid from palm oil to L-ascorbic acid. The resulting chemical bond creates a fat-soluble compound that contains vitamin C.

Ascorbyl palmitate protects the critical cell membranes in skin. Esters like ascorbyl palmitate should be the vitamin C forms of choice for skin care products because they are absorbed and retained by the skin substantially better than L-ascorbic acid.

Scurvy: Not Just in Sailors

Vitamin C deficiencies are much more common than many doctors believe. In 1997, a University of Arizona team led by researcher Carol Johnston, Ph.D., tested blood samples from a random group of 494 middle-income people. The tests showed that 30 percent were vitamin C depleted, and that 6.3 percent suffered from the more severe condition called vitamin C deficiency, which produces the symptoms of the disease once called scurvy, that afflicted sailors and others deprived of fresh fruits and vegetables for long periods.

Vitamin C is the foundation of my antioxidant program, but it is also a fragile, unstable nutrient. Since the vitamin C levels in our foods are affected by climate, soil conditions, storage time, temperature, and cooking, it is impossible to tell exactly how much vitamin C you are actually getting at mealtime—hence the wisdom of taking 500 to 1000 mg of supplemental vitamin C a day.

Vitamin C (L-Ascorbic Acid and Ascorbyl Palmitate)

Vitamin C is ascorbic acid, a water-soluble compound. Ascorbyl palmitate is ascorbic acid bonded to a fatty acid to make a fat-soluble delivery system for vitamin C.

FEATURES AND BENEFITS
- Water-soluble (L-ascorbic acid) or fat-soluble (vitamin C esters like ascorbyl palmitate)
- Promotes collagen production
- Essential for functioning of neurotransmitters, including dopamine, serotonin, and acetylcholine
- Accumulates inside white blood cells to maintain strong immune response
- Defends against free radicals in the skin created by sunlight, ozone, and harsh chemicals
- Accumulates in the central nervous system to fight free radical activity

SYMPTOMS AND EFFECTS OF A VITAMIN C DEFICIENCY
- Scurvy (spongy, bleeding gums; bleeding under the skin; extreme weakness)
- Parkinson's disease
- Loss of muscle tone
- Loss of sense of well-being
- Wrinkles
- Weakened immunity; increased susceptibility to infections

INTAKE REQUIREMENTS AND SUPPLEMENT RECOMMENDATIONS
- RDI: 60 mg
- No observed adverse effects level: 1000 mg or more
- Wrinkle-Free recommendation: 1,000 mg ascorbic acid and 500 mg ascorbyl palmitate

The RDI of 60 mg is inadequate to provide the antioxidant action that vitamin C offers or to maintain reasonable levels in skin tissues. Even if you take the higher oral doses I recommend, you will need to use cosmetics that contain a vitamin C ester such as ascorbyl palmitate to attain vitamin C skin levels high enough to reduce inflammation effectively.

To avoid gastric discomfort and maintain adequate blood levels, divide the dosage into three or four portions a day.

For maximum absorption of the ascorbic acid form, look for capsules of vitamin C, or add powdered vitamin C crystals to water or tea. (Hard vitamin C tablets tend to pass through the digestive tract intact) Note: There is good evidence that vitamin C is better absorbed when it is combined with bioflavonoids (anti-inflammatory antioxidants found in citrus fruits and other foods). However, vitamin C products with bioflavonoids do not contain enough of them to produce this effect.

The makers of Ester-C® (which, despite its name, is not a true vitamin C ester) also make superior-absorption claims for their mineral-bound vitamin C product, which also contains vitamin C metabolites (breakdown products). While Ester-C® has shown superior absorption in rats and in isolated human cells, the only peer-reviewed human clinical trial showed no absorption advantage. Both Ester-C® and vitamin C with bioflavonoids are substantially more costly than plain L-ascorbic acid—a fact that would seem to cancel out any moderate increase in bodily absorption or cellular uptake these products may offer.

NONINFLAMMATORY FOOD SOURCES

- Broccoli
- Cantaloupe
- Citrus fruits
- Red bell peppers
- Strawberries
- Tomatoes

Vitamin E: Every Cell's "Perimeter Defense"

Vitamin E is composed of eight separate components, which are divided into two groups, four tocopherols and four tocotrienols. To get all the available benefits, I recommend a "combination" vitamin E supplement that offers a mix of tocotrienols and tocopherols—especially gamma tocopherols.

FEATURES AND BENEFITS

- Fat-soluble
- Lowers cholesterol

- Reduces blood pressure
- Prevents cataracts
- Decreases risk of stroke
- Enhances immune system
- Decreases symptoms of Alzheimer's disease
- Prevents heart attacks
- Protects cell plasma membrane

NONINFLAMMATORY FOOD SOURCES
- Almonds
- Asparagus
- Hazelnuts
- Olives
- Pecans
- Spinach
- Sunflower seeds

INTAKE REQUIREMENTS AND SUPPLEMENT RECOMMENDATIONS
- RDI: 30 IU
- No observed adverse effects level: 1,200 IU
- Wrinkle-Free recommendation: 400 to 800 IU

Look for soft gel capsules that contain a total of 400 to 800 IU of vitamin E. Because it is fat soluble, take it with meals for greatest absorption.

Minerals

Calcium

With so many women (and an increasing number of men) concerned about bone density, calcium and magnesium are very important minerals. Nothing is more aging than the dowager's hump and bent spine of advanced osteoporosis or the fragility that results from paper-thin bones. Your mother used to tell you to drink your milk for strong bones, but supplements will also do the trick. As we get older bone density decreases, and I strongly recommend calcium supplementation.

A debate continues over the best form of calcium to take. It all comes down to price. Chelated forms (for example, calcium citrate or malate) are absorbed by the body a bit better but are also noticeably costlier than calcium carbonate—the standard, cheapest form. Calcium carbonate is a good choice unless your digestive system is weak. If it is, take a chelated version or increase your calcium carbonate intake to account for the lowered absorption level.

FEATURES AND BENEFITS
- Essential for healthy teeth, gums, and bones
- Reduces cholesterol deposits
- Relieves muscle spasms
- Lowers blood pressure
- Relieves PMS in some cases
- Assists in absorption of nutrients across cell membranes
- Aids muscle contraction
- Facilitates nerve conduction

SYMPTOMS AND EFFECTS OF A CALCIUM DEFICIENCY
- Osteoporosis
- Bleeding gums
- Rickets

NONINFLAMMATORY FOOD SOURCES
- Collards, kale, and turnip greens
- Cooked broccoli (cooking makes the calcium more available)
- Low-fat yogurt
- Nuts and seeds
- Sardines or salmon (canned with bones)
- Sea vegetables (dulse, kelp, etc.)
- Tofu
- Wheat germ

INTAKE REQUIREMENTS AND SUPPLEMENT RECOMMENDATIONS
- RDI: 1,000
- No observed adverse effects level: 1,500 mg
- Wrinkle-Free recommendation: 1,200 mg

The richest food sources of calcium are sea vegetables (highest concentration per ounce), cheese, and tofu. Milk and milk products (except yogurt) are the next richest sources, but I do not recommend them as primary calcium sources for my adult patients, since they tend to promote inflammation and are difficult for many people to digest. Further, to meet the RDA standards, you need to consume at least three eight-ounce glasses of milk or more than five ounces of hard cheese a day—a goal that can be difficult for many adults. Plain yogurt, greens, seeds, and nuts are better choices but must also be consumed in large quantities to reach the RDA levels, so supplementation is a logical strategy for securing adequate daily calcium. I never recommend calcium without its nutritional partner, magnesium.

Chromium

FEATURES AND BENEFITS
- Regulates blood sugar levels
- Helps metabolize body fat
- Lowers cholesterol
- Helps regulate insulin
- Promotes weight loss
- Important in the metabolism of carbohydrates and fats
- Helps to regulate the amount of glucose in the blood
- Is needed for insulin to work properly

SYMPTOMS AND EFFECTS OF A CHROMIUM DEFICIENCY
- Impaired glucose tolerance
- Impaired growth

NONINFLAMMATORY FOOD SOURCES
- Brewer's yeast
- Calves Liver

INTAKE REQUIREMENTS AND SUPPLEMENT RECOMMENDATIONS
- RDI: 120 mcg
- No observed adverse effects level: 1,000 mg
- Wrinkle-Free recommendation: 200 mcg chromium polynicotinate

It is estimated that up to one third of Americans do not consume these minimal levels, given the unpopularity of the two best food sources. I recommend taking 200 mcg of chromium polynicotinate as a supplement daily. (I do not recommend taking chromium in the form of chromium picolinate, which is associated with some safety concerns.)

> **Quick Tip:** Take chromium the same time as vitamin C to maximize absorption.

Magnesium

FEATURES AND BENEFITS
- Regulates blood pressure
- Promotes muscle tone
- Aids healthy bone and tooth development
- Needed for energy production and protein synthesis
- Counteracts negative effects of stress hormones

SYMPTOMS AND EFFECTS OF A MAGNESIUM DEFICIENCY
- Muscle spasms
- Tremor
- Convulsions
- Mental derangement

NONINFLAMMATORY FOOD SOURCES
- Almonds
- Avocados
- Dried soybeans
- Oatmeal (not instant)
- Peanuts
- Tofu

INTAKE REQUIREMENTS AND SUPPLEMENT RECOMMENDATIONS
- RDI: 400 mg
- No observed adverse effects level: 700 mg
- Wrinkle-Free recommendation: half to equal amounts of magnesium to calcium; 600 to 1,200 mg depending on calcium intake

Keep in mind that cooking can dissolve as much as three quarters of the available mineral, causing it to leach into the pan.

Selenium
FEATURES AND BENEFITS
- Essential in formation of glutathione
- Neutralizes poisons like mercury and arsenic
- Cuts the rate of certain cancers
- Provides anti-inflammatory relief from psoriasis and rheumatoid arthritis
- Protects cells against the effects of free radicals
- Prevents oxidation of unsaturated fatty acids
- Helps with proper heart function
- Needed for proper immune function

NONINFLAMMATORY FOOD SOURCES
- Brazil nuts
- Garlic
- Liver, such as calves liver
- Poultry
- Seafood, both fish and shellfish

INTAKE REQUIREMENTS AND SUPPLEMENT RECOMMENDATIONS
- RDI: 70 mcg
- No observed adverse effects level: 200 mcg
- Wrinkle-Free recommendation: 200 mcg

Zinc
FEATURES AND BENEFITS
- Helps heal wounds
- Boosts energy metabolism

- Helps body maintain healthy collagen
- An element of superoxidismutase (SOD), a key free radical fighter
- Essential for normal cell division

SYMPTOMS AND EFFECTS OF A ZINC DEFICIENCY
- Worsening of acne, psoriasis, and eczema

NONINFLAMMATORY FOOD SOURCES
- Brazil nuts
- Chicken
- Halibut
- Oatmeal (not instant)
- Salmon
- Sunflower seeds
- Turkey

INTAKE REQUIREMENTS AND SUPPLEMENT RECOMMENDATIONS
- RDI: 15 mg
- No observed adverse effects level: 30 mg
- Wrinkle-Free recommendation: 15 to 30 mg

Amino Acids and Nutritional Isolates

The final group of recommended supplements is a mix of antioxidants and nutritional compounds. For some, there are no existing RDAs. I have derived supplement recommendations from published research sources.

L-Carnitine
FEATURES AND BENEFITS
- Allows fats to be transported into the mitochondria for energy
- Promotes weight loss by improving fat metabolism
- Prevents free radical damage

Symptoms and effects of an L-carnitine deficiency
- Inability to harvest the energy stored in fatty acids and a buildup of fatty intermediates that can prove toxic to cells

Noninflammatory food sources
- Dairy products
- Meat

Intake requirements and supplement recommendations
- RDI: None established
- No observed adverse effects level: None established
- Wrinkle-Free recommendation: 500 to 1,500 mg, depending on age and health. If you are under thirty years old and feel energetic, you will do well on 500 mg. If you have chronic health problems, such as diabetes, heart disease, or chronic fatigue, I would advise you to take between 1,000 to 1,500 mg. For maximum absorption, divide the doses into three separate portions.

Acetyl L-Carnitine

Another form of carnitine, called acetyl L-carnitine is available as a supplement. It cannot be derived from food. When scientists add the acetyl portion to the carnitine, it allows the carnitine to pass the blood-brain barrier more readily. Acetyl L-carnitine is therapeutic to brain cells. I have found in my clinical practice that supplementing diets with acetyl L-carnitine tends to accelerate fat loss much better in my patients than L-carnitine alone.

Features and benefits
- Improves cognitive function, including memory and problem-solving ability
- Promotes skin health

Intake requirements and supplement recommendations
- RDI: None established
- No observed adverse effects level: None established

- Wrinkle-Free recommendation: 500 to 1,000 mg. Sources of acetyl L-carnitine can be found in Appendix B.

Coenzyme Q 10 (CoQ10)

FEATURES AND BENEFITS

- Fat soluble
- Relieves congestive heart failure
- Reduces angina and high blood pressure
- Increases metabolic efficiency to fight weight gain
- Reduces risk of breast and prostate cancer
- Preserves the antioxidant action of vitamin C
- May prevent atherosclerosis
- Protects both the mitochondria and the cell membrane against oxidative damage
- Strengthens the gums to protect against periodontal disease

SYMPTOMS AND EFFECTS OF A COENZYME Q 10 DEFICIENCY

- CoQ10 deficiency is common in individuals with heart disease. Heart tissue biopsies performed on patients with different types of heart diseases showed a coenzyme Q 10 deficiency in 50 to 75 percent of the cases.
- CoQ10 deficiency can affect brain and nerve function

NONINFLAMMATORY FOOD SOURCES

Only small amounts of CoQ10 are available in foods. You would have to eat a pound of sardines or two and a half pounds of peanuts to get the minimum daily amount recommended for healthy people. CoQ10 is best taken as a supplement, and optimal absorption occurs when it is taken with meals. (Note: If you have heart problems, check with your physician for the right dosage of CoQ10 for you.)

INTAKE REQUIREMENTS AND SUPPLEMENT RECOMMENDATIONS

- RDI: None established
- No observed adverse effects level: None established—considered extremely safe for healthy persons even at high doses. While it

may be beneficial for diabetes or heart disease, individuals with these conditions should not take CoQ10 except under a doctor's supervision.

- Wrinkle-Free recommendation: 30 to 300 mg

CoQ10 levels tend to drop as you grow older, particularly in postmenopausal women. Since CoQ10 is essential for heart health, some cardiologists believe that the increased incidence of congestive heart failure in women of this age is due in part to the significant drop in their CoQ10 levels.

Glutamine

FEATURES AND BENEFITS

- Heals gastrointestinal tract irritation
- Aids in treating individuals with gastrointestinal diseases, such as Crohn's disease, colitis, short bowel syndrome, and irritable bowel syndrome, who require higher levels of glutamine
- Reduces fatigue
- Increases endurance during exercise
- Helps counteract the effects of alcoholism
- Raises serum glucose levels to fight hypoglycemia
- Aids the liver and the intestines
- Strengthens the immune system
- Preserves muscle tissue
- Growth hormone release
- Serves as fuel for the heart muscle
- Aids in glutathione production in the cells

NONINFLAMMATORY FOOD SOURCES

- Fish
- Legumes
- Poultry

- RDI: None established
- No observed adverse effects level: None established
- Wrinkle-Free recommendation: 1,500 mg (500 mg three times a day). Check Appendix B for sources of glutamine.

Levels of this protective amino acid fall sharply as you age and during any illness, burn, or trauma. It is especially helpful for athletes and the aging population. I recommend higher levels for athletes, aging patients, and those who are suffering from acute and chronic diseases. It is extremely effective in healing the GI tract.

OPC (Grape Seed Extract/Pycnogenol)

OPC is the scientific name of an antioxidant complex derived from various plants—especially grape seeds and pine bark. OPC stands for oligomeric proanthocyanidin—a class of extremely potent antioxidant compounds. Many experts believe that the OPCs in red wine explain the French paradox—that is, that the French enjoy relatively low rates of heart disease despite a diet high in saturated fat. OPCs are believed to help prevent the oxidation of blood fats and cholesterol upon which much arterial heart disease is blamed.

OPCs are important to skin care because they protect collagen from free radicals, dampen inflammation, and help maintain the health and integrity of blood vessels. As years go by, capillaries and veins become fragile, resulting in a decline in blood circulation. (In France, grape seed OPC is an approved prescription drug for treating weak blood vessels.) Preserving the blood vessels improves oxygen and food delivery to skin cells, which stimulates their growth and repair.

Consumers can easily become confused by the terminology and competing claims surrounding the two leading supplemental sources of OPCs: grape seed extract and pine bark extract. I recommend taking OPCs in the form of grape seed extract, because the OPC complex found in grape seeds appears to substantially exceed the antioxidant power of the OPC complex found in pine bark. Note: Pine bark extracts are often referred to as "pycnogenol"—the original scientific term for OPCs. However, the term "pycnogenol" is out of common scientific use and is now the registered trademark of a proprietary pine bark extract (Pycnogenol). To avoid confusion, most researchers use the generic term OPC when discussing the antioxidant complexes found in grape seeds and pine bark.

OPCs are also found in berries, grapes, cherries, and wine. OPCs are the main precursors of the blue-violet and red pigments in plants (anthocyanins). Look for reddish-purple capsules to be sure you are getting a concentrated natural product.

FEATURES AND BENEFITS
- Blocks the key enzymes that degrade collagen and other connective tissues
- Neutralizes xanthine oxidase (major generator of free radicals), the potent hydroxyl free radical, and prevents oxidation of body fats and cholesterol
- Now believed to be the key factor in the cardiovascular health–promoting powers of red wine

INTAKE REQUIREMENTS AND SUPPLEMENT RECOMMENDATIONS
- RDI: None established
- No observed adverse effects level: None established
- Wrinkle-Free recommendation: 30 to 100 mg

GLA (Gamma Linolenic Acid)

GLA is an omega-6 essential fatty acid. It is rapidly converted to dihomo-gamma-linolenic acid, the precursor of prostaglandin E1, a potent anti-inflammatory agent. We become deficient in GLA when large amounts of sugar, trans fatty acids (margarine, hydrogenated oils), and red meats and dairy products are consumed, or when levels of delta-6 desaturase are low or absent.

Very little GLA is found in the average western diet. Borage oil is the richest supplemental source (17 to 25 percent GLA), followed by black currant oil (15 to 20 percent GLA) and evening primrose oil (EPO) (7 to 10 percent GLA). Borage and evening primrose oils are the most common supplemental sources. GLA should be taken with food, to increase absorption.

FEATURES AND BENEFITS
- Production of prostaglandins
- Prevents hardening of the arteries
- Lowers cholesterol
- Lowers blood pressure
- Inhibits blood clotting
- Reduces blood triglycerides
- Reduces LDL cholesterol levels
- Prevents blockage of arteries
- Enhances die-off of cancer cells
- Suppresses growth of malignant tumors
- Offsets degenerative signs of aging
- May help PMS (weak evidence)
- Reduces benign breast disease, eczema, psoriasis, obesity, and vascular disorders
- Effective to varying degrees in treating arthritis, alcoholism, asthma, diabetic neuropathy, and multiple sclerosis

INTAKE REQUIREMENTS AND SUPPLEMENT RECOMMENDATIONS
- RDI: None established
- No observed adverse effects level: None established
- Wrinkle-Free recommendation: 250 to 1,000 mg

Turmeric

This brilliant yellow spice has been used as a culinary mainstay in many cultures for thousands of years. Turmeric, a member of the ginger family, is the ingredient that gives Asian curries their characteristic bright-yellow hue. The spice's active compounds are potent anti-inflammatory antioxidant substances called curcuminoids.

FEATURES AND BENEFITS
- Prevents free radical formation and neutralizes existing free radicals
- May reduce risk of Alzheimer's disease
- Antiviral, noninflammatory, anticancer effects

- Lowers bad cholesterol
- Treats AIDS by blocking activation of the LTR gene in the HIV DNA
- Used in India's ancient ayurvedic medicine as a stomach tonic, for cuts, wounds, poor vision, rheumatic pains, coughs, liver disease, and to increase milk production
- Protects the liver

INTAKE REQUIREMENTS AND SUPPLEMENT RECOMMENDATIONS
- RDI: None established
- No observed adverse effects level: None established
- Wrinkle-Free recommendation: 250 to 1,000 mg

Turmeric should be stored in the freezer or refrigerator to keep the volatile oils fresh and active.

Wrinkle-Free Daily Supplements

We have reviewed the supplements that will fight inflammation in your body, raise your energy, and retard aging. What follows is a schedule of supplements you are to take each day on the Perricone Wrinkle-Free Program.

This program will benefit anyone, but will work especially well if you are in generally good health. For my patients who suffer from chronic illnesses or are extremely low on energy, I tailor special plans.

Take the nutrients in these recommended doses.

Always check with your physician before taking new supplements.

BREAKFAST
- Multivitamin (make sure this contains at least 2,500 IU of vitamin A in the carotenoid form, but no more than 10,000 mg)
- B complex—choose a formula providing at least the RDA for each B vitamin
- Vitamin C (ascorbic acid)—500 mg

- Vitamin C ester—500 mg ascorbyl palmitate (not Ester-C®)
- Vitamin E—200 to 400 mg (tocopherol-tocotrienol blend)
- Alpha lipoic acid—50 mg
- Calcium—1,000 mg
- Magnesium—400 mg
- Chromium—200 mcg (choose chromium polynicotinate)
- Selenium—200 mcg
- L-carnitine—500 to 1,000 mg
- Acetyl L-carnitine—500 mg
- Coenzyme Q10—15 to 150 mg
- Grape seed extract (OPCs)—30 to 100 mg
- Turmeric—250 mg
- L-glutamine—250 to 1,000 mg
- Omega-3 fatty acids (fish, flax, hemp oil)—2,000 mg
- GLA (Omega-6 fatty acids) (borage or evening primrose oil)—
  250 to 1,000 mg

LUNCH
- Vitamin C (ascorbic acid)—500 mg
- Alpha lipoic acid—50 mg
- Acetyl L-carnitine—500 mg
- Coenzyme Q 10—15 to 150 mg
- L-glutamine—250 to 1,000 mg
- Omega-3 fatty acids (fish, flax or hemp oil)—2,000 mg
- GLA (Omega-6 fatty acid) (borage or evening primrose oil)—250
  to 1,000 mg

Extreme Measures (or, Glutathione to the Rescue!)

Warren has been a patient of mine for a number of years. A forty-year-old college professor, he has been HIV positive for the past ten years. Warren has been fortunate; he has never devel-

continued on next page

oped the symptoms of AIDS, and his T-cell count remains normal. Warren recently called to say that he was experiencing extreme fatigue. He was so exhausted he could not go to work—in fact, he could not even get out of bed in the morning.

Warren had consulted his internal medicine physician. His laboratory work came back satisfactory. He was also checked for other problems, including heart disease and infections such as tuberculosis. Again, all these test results were negative. Yet Warren was still exhausted.

One of the hallmarks of HIV infection is that it is pro-inflammatory, a state that leads to a reduction of antioxidants in the body with an increase in stress hormones such as cortisol. Glutathione, the body's own endogenous antioxidant defense system, is often severely depleted. I explained to Warren that since his physical exam and laboratory studies were normal, we would try to elevate his cellular glutathione levels by adding some new supplements to his regimen. For years, Warren had been following a good multivitamin program. We now needed to do more. I added three new supplements to Warren's usual regimen and increased the levels of certain antioxidants he was already taking.

The first supplement I introduced was N-acetyl-cysteine, an amino acid that is an antioxidant and a precursor of glutathione. I asked him to take 1,000 mg twice daily. In addition, I recommended that he begin taking glutamine powder, another amino acid. Glutamine is a precursor of glutathione as well, but it also acts as a powerful anti-inflammatory and enhances the body's nutritional status. I suggested a dose of a half teaspoon of pure glutamine powder three times daily. Finally, I asked him to increase his alpha lipoic acid intake to 250 mg twice daily.

I also provided Warren with a glutathione cream in a highly penetrating base that I had recently developed. One of the problems we face in keeping our glutathione at optimum levels is finding the most effective delivery system to the body. Glutathione cannot be taken orally, because it is a tripeptide that is digested. Prior to my invention of a transdermal glutathione cream, the only effective method of getting glutathione into the body was intravenously, and that is not very practical. I started Warren on the cream, which contains 450 mg per cubic centimeter (cc) of glutathione. I instructed him to place 1 cc on each of his forearms three times a day, rubbing his forearms together to promote absorption of the glutathione.

I called Warren approximately four to five days later and reached his answering machine. I worried that he may have become so weak he could not even answer his phone. To calm my rising concern, I called one of his coworkers at the university and was informed that he was in his office. A few minutes later, Warren's strong voice was assuring me that he felt terrific and had resumed his normal work schedule. I was gratified that we had managed to elevate the glutathione level in his cells, which quickly restored his energy level.

Treatment with transdermal delivery of glutathione should be routine practice for anyone suffering from any illness characterized by extreme fatigue, since glutathione levels will drop whenever inflammation is present. Since many of my patients are under stress—whether work related, from personal problems, or as a result of common cold or flu—I have them take the supplements I recommended to Warren. In many cases I also recommend the topical glutathione to patients who are severely fatigued or stressed.

Now that you are aware of the nutrients and supplements you need to consume on the Perricone Wrinkle-Free Program, it's time to tell you how to fight inflammation from the outside by using the latest, scientifically developed skin care products on your face and body. You have seen how nutrition can reduce inflammation; the topicals are even more exciting, are easy to obtain and use, and are a delightful way to pamper your skin.

5

Topical Anti-inflammatories for Reversing and Preventing Signs of Aging

Whether you care for your skin with soap and water or the most extravagantly packaged creams and lotions, there is always room for improvement in your complexion. So far in *The Perricone Prescription,* you have learned how to nourish your body with foods and supplements that will quell the inflammation that ages you from within. In this chapter, I will introduce you to a number of breakthroughs involving antioxidant anti-inflammatories that are applied to the skin and absorbed into the cells where they can repair damage and rejuvenate your skin.

You have no doubt heard about the "secret ingredients" that promise cellular repair in so many skin care products today. I have discovered, researched, tested, formulated, and patented a number of supernutrients for your skin. Scientifically proven compounds like vitamin C ester, alpha lipoic acid, and tocotrienol (a powerful form of vitamin E) are revolutionizing the way we care for our skin. I have been working with other substances you may not have heard of, including DMAE and PPC (polyenylphosphatidyl choline). I will use a number of case histories to illustrate and explain how these antioxidants work miracles.

You will learn the optimal skin care program for your entire body, including the face, hands, legs, which are subject to so much abuse. Whether your skin is normal, dry, or oily, the antiaging revolution in skin care will work for you. I will recommend what topicals you should use to make your skin dewy, clear, and even. Since I prefer to approach skin care according to skin color, I will discuss the characteristics of Northern European, African-American, Mediterranean, Asian, and Latino skin, the problems you are likely to have, and the right products to use on your particular type of skin.

While we are on the subject of topicals, I would wager that many of you would like to know about the effectiveness of cellulite creams and massage oils. Let me tell you Shelley's story and how her own program of skin care did more harm than good.

Too Much of a Good Thing

As I dropped off a chart at the front desk in my office, I noticed an attractive, blond woman in her late thirties sitting in the reception area. She was noticeably anxious.

"That's Shelley," my office manager whispered. "She looks like she didn't get here a minute too soon." Even from across the room, I could see that a bright red rash covered her face and neck. It was no wonder she appeared so stressed.

I walked Shelley to the examination room. No sooner had we finished shaking hands than Shelley asked me about starting an antiaging program as soon as possible. To my surprise, she expressed no concern about her rash. In fact, she did not even mention it. Shelley had recently broken up with her longtime boyfriend and was up for a partnership in a top law firm. She wanted to look fabulous as she embarked on a new life. Though her long working hours were instrumental in helping her advance in her career, she did not want them to show on her face.

Shelley had created her own skin care regimen, an amalgam of Retin-A, a prescription cream with wrinkle-fighting benefits; alpha- and beta-hydroxy creams; and a vitamin C serum made from L-ascorbic acid. In addition, Shelley used a combination apricot hull–oatmeal scrub for cleansing, and used a loofah instead of a face cloth. Twice a week she "treated" herself to a clay mask facial. I listened in growing horror and disbelief. Shelley had not left out a single topical proinflammatory substance I could think of. I was surprised that the rash wasn't much worse. As I examined her face and neck, I gave her a course in Skin 101 in the hope that she would realize that skin care and furniture refinishing have nothing in common.

Getting the Red Out

Shelley's natural complexion was the peaches-and-cream type enjoyed by many natural blondes. At the moment I met her, though, her skin resembled another fruit—overripe strawberries. Shelley needed some serious help in treating her rash. My first task at hand was to calm the skin and return it to a noninflammatory state. Topical vitamin C was my first treatment for Shelley. Fortunately, I was able to reach into my medical cabinet and take out a jar of concentrated vitamin C cream. It had not always been so. My efforts toward developing such a cream had begun years earlier in medical school.

Vitamin C to the Rescue

One bright, sunny August morning, I had taken a particularly long run. By late afternoon, my face had turned bright red from painful sunburn. It occurred to me that since vitamin C was a powerful antioxidant, perhaps it would also act as an anti-inflammatory to help resolve the burn more rapidly. That night, I made a vitamin C solution by mixing crushed vitamin C tablets in water and patted it on my face. At first it stung, but the discomfort soon subsided and I was able to sleep. In the morning, the burn was definitely better. The swelling and redness had greatly diminished, although they had not disappeared entirely. Yet my shoulders, on which I hadn't applied the vitamin C, were still quite red and tender. My vitamin C solution showed potential, but there was still work to be done.

Several years later, I returned to the use of vitamin C with a new approach. I reasoned that the solubility of the vitamin C molecule (L-ascorbic acid) interfered with its anti-inflammatory effects. Ascorbic acid, the natural form of vitamin C, is water soluble. Ascorbic acid cannot penetrate the surface of the skin, which repels water-soluble substances. The acidity of the vitamin C also diminished the anti-inflammatory effects. Ascorbic acid lives up to its name. It is very acidic, which can be irritating to the skin. Then there is the problem of potency. Ascorbic acid is fragile and unstable, and it breaks down rapidly. When formulated into a solution, ascorbic acid loses its strength within twenty-four hours. I set out to find a form of vitamin C that would be nonirritating, fat soluble, and retain its strength in skin care preparations.

Vitamin C Ester

My search led me to a compound known as vitamin C ester. It is composed of the basic vitamin C molecule (L-ascorbic acid) joined with palmitic acid, a fatty acid derived from palm oil. Vitamin C ester is completely nonirritating and can even be used on an open cut without stinging. This in itself was a leap from the burning and irritation caused by topical ascorbic acid. More important, vitamin C ester is fat soluble, easing its absorption by the skin and the cell plasma membrane.

The antioxidant power of vitamin C ester at the cell plasma membrane provides key protection at a critical time. Research done by Procter & Gamble scientists found that vitamin C ester is absorbed more quickly and achieves six to seven times higher levels in the skin than ascorbic acid.

I tried vitamin C ester formulations on sunburns. This time, I got the results I had been looking for years earlier in my simple ascorbic acid experiment. Using a UV lamp, I created small sunburns on the forearms of test subjects. I supplied half the group with a cream containing vitamin C ester, and gave the other half the same cream without the fortification of the antioxidant vitamin. Within a day, the burns treated with vitamin C ester were less red. Those treated with the other cream stayed red for days.

Today, my patients use vitamin C ester–fortified cream at night to repair the damage inflicted by the daily doses of free radicals in their environment and diet. I have treated patients who have spent twenty years enjoying outdoor activities without sun protection whose faces now show premature lines, wrinkles, and discoloration. After using vitamin C ester for thirty days, the change was remarkable. Their skin glowed, and the crow's-feet diminished and in some cases actually disappeared.

Vitamin C Ester

Function
Proven antioxidant anti-inflammatory that helps to prevent free radical damage in all environments.

Characteristics
Lipid soluble, neutral pH, nonacidic, thus nonirritating and nonstinging. Solubility enables this form of vitamin C to penetrate the surface of the skin rapidly in amounts greater than can be achieved by water soluble vitamin C (L-ascorbic acid).

Benefits
· Provides readily available form of vitamin C to the skin
· Can be used by those with sensitive skin
· Helps to protect from damage by free radicals and inflammation

Shelley was a prime candidate for vitamin C ester. For her, the results were transformative. The vitamin C ester cream got rid of her rash, and also within a few weeks many of the fine lines on her face had diminished. Her skin, which had a dry, almost papery texture resulting from her blond heritage and many summers at the beach, was actually thickening and plumping up again. Her face had begun to glow, the hallmark of the power of vitamin C ester to improve skin tone and texture and rebuild and repair the natural collagen dramatically.

After a few months of applying vitamin C ester cream at night, Shelley's skin improved so much that she no longer needed to wear makeup during the day, and she happily abandoned the idea of expensive laser treatments.

It's Never Too Late

I saw dramatic evidence of vitamin C ester's ability to thicken atrophic, or thin skin, the result of years of damage from the sun, in the treatment of an elderly patient. A seventy-five-year-old man came to my office with his father, who, at ninety-five, had severe skin problems. The father had worked outside all his life, and now that he was retired, enjoyed spending time in his garden. His skin had become so paper thin that merely brushing the back of his hand or forearm against furniture caused the skin to tear and bleed. Dermatologists see this kind of problem regularly in older people who have suffered from photo damage. At one time, the standard treatment was to apply topical moisturizers and to avoid sun exposure. Now that I had vitamin C ester, I knew I had more to offer this patient.

Since the patient had a large body surface area that needed to be treated, I instructed my compounding pharmacist to prepare one-pound jars of vitamin C ester (ascorbyl palmitate) at a 10 percent level in a moisturizing base. I instructed the patient and his son to apply the vitamin C ester cream to the entire body once daily, and to the problem areas (the face, neck, and forearms) twice daily. I explained it would take some time before they would see any improvement, given his skin's fragility. I asked the patient to schedule an appointment a few months later.

Sunscreen as a Habit

All skin tones are vulnerable to damage from the sun's ultraviolet rays. Applying sunscreen at the start of your day should be as automatic as combing your hair. If your skin is oily, use oil-

continued on next page

free sunscreens that will not clog your pores. Many moisturizers have built-in sun protection, as noted by the SPF (sun protection factor) rating. Just make sure that any product you use has an SPF *no lower than 15.*

Following is an abbreviated list of the companies making the best sunscreens:

- Avon—Sunseekers
- Beiersdorf—Eucerin Daily Sun Defense
- Estée Lauder—In the Sun products
- Fisher Pharmaceuticals—Ultrasol
- Hawaiian Tropic—Suncare
- Procter & Gamble—Olay UV Protective lotions
- Schering-Plough—Coppertone products
- Sun Pharmaceutical—Banana Boat products
- Westwood-Squibb—PreSun products

Approximately ten weeks after the first visit, my patient's son called. He was quite excited. To their amazement, his father's skin was no longer tearing or breaking, and it looked to him as if his skin had visibly thickened. I was delighted that the results had been achieved faster than I had expected. I looked forward to seeing the older man at his second visit.

When he returned at the three-month point, his skin was much more supple. The signs of thin skin had diminished; there was no longer tearing or bleeding. Many of the other symptoms of this problem (black-and-blue marks on the skin, for example) had also diminished greatly. I was pleased by this demonstration of the powerful abilities of vitamin C ester to repair skin that had both damaged collagen and elastin.

Alpha Lipoic Acid

As much as I study and do research, I find my best source of new discoveries is my patients. My experience with Lauren was a case of the pupil teaching the teacher. She was thirty-five years old when she first came to my office. She had suffered for years from rosacea, a condition most commonly found in women, in which the blood vessels under the face swell, causing persistent redness of the skin. Her condition had progressed to the point where the small blood vessels of the face had enlarged and had begun to show through the skin; little red lines, similar to routes on a map, were visible.

Small pink bumps were also present. Lauren was understandably dismayed by the condition of her skin. Rosacea can be notoriously difficult to treat. In fact, scientists have not identified the cause, though varying theories exist. No one disputes that whatever the cause, serious subcutaneous and cutaneous inflammation are present.

Lauren admitted that for years she had used only water to wash her face. She believed the common myth that washing with water only will keep facial skin moist and will stave off wrinkles. That is a terrible misconception. If you do not clean your skin, bacteria and other pathogens build up. These bacteria can lead to all kinds of dermatological and general health problems. I explained to Lauren that many of my patients who tell me they have cleaned their faces with only water for years have rosacea.

There is evidence that rosacea may be caused by organisms living in the sebaceous, oil-rich areas of the skin. I am opposed to using only water, cold cream, or a similar agent to clean your face. I do not recommend using a harsh cleanser, because that results in dryness and inflammation. Fortunately, there are many excellent products available that will thoroughly cleanse your face and remove any buildup of bacteria or pathogens. A list of good cleansers appears on page 132.

I started Lauren on oral and topical antibiotics because of the severity of her rosacea. In addition, I gave her a nutritive cleanser containing alpha lipoic acid, instructing her to cleanse her face thoroughly each morning and evening. I also gave her a high-potency alpha lipoic acid lotion, and told her to apply it to her entire face and neck twice a day. Alpha lipoic acid (ALA), the universal antioxidant, is both water and fat soluble. This means that ALA is easily absorbed through the lipid layers of the skin and works equally well as a free radical fighter in both the cell plasma membrane and in the watery interior of the cell.

As I examined the rest of Lauren's face, I noted that she had significant edema around the eyes. The puffiness made her look older than her years. I observed that aside from the redness of her cheeks and nose, the rest of her face looked dull and lifeless; her skin lacked vibrancy. I asked Lauren about her lifestyle, diet, and exercise habits. She admitted that she was undergoing a particularly stressful time in her life. She was a journalist with a top-tier news daily. Although she loved her work, hers was a career filled with deadlines and pressures, currently made even more intense as her paper was temporarily shorthanded. Lauren had to do twice the work in half the time. It was obvious that Lauren's stress levels were out of control.

Her dietary routine started with a breakfast consisting of a bagel and coffee snatched from a kiosk at the train station. She normally gulped down a fruit smoothie for lunch on her way to the gym for a workout. Since Lauren was bringing home a briefcase full of work each night, dinner had to be quick and easy. She usually microwaved a large potato, which she topped with a tablespoon of low-fat yogurt. I cringed as I listened to the abuse she was unwittingly heaping on her body. Where was the protein? How could her cells rebuild and repair themselves? Where were the essential fatty acids to nourish her brain, lower stress hormones, hold her moods on an even keel, and keep her skin moist and plumped up? Lauren also looked dehydrated. She told me she rarely drank water—another reason for her gray pallor. There were some antioxidants in the fruit smoothie, but not enough to combat the high-glycemic impact of the bagel, the sugar in the smoothie, and the potato.

Lauren proudly reported that she did not have a sweet tooth and never ate candy or cookies or drank soda—but she had no idea how quickly that bagel and potato were turning into sugar in her bloodstream. If you refer to a glycemic index you will see how high both these foods are on the glycemic scale. Foods high on the glycemic index are proven to accelerate aging in your body and take a terrible toll on your skin. A burst of inflammation that results from a rapid rise in blood sugar occurs in all your cells, especially in your skin cells.

At the same time, water metabolism changes. This is why Lauren's eyes were puffy and she was losing the contours in her face. Perhaps nothing makes us look our age quite as much as tired, drooping eyelids and saggy, baggy skin under the eyes. The high glycemic foods were caus-ing her to retain fluids in the skin cells. And let's not forget that long-term elevation of blood sugar leads to glycation—a state you want to avoid if you want resilient, unlined skin.

I put Lauren on a vitamin C ester serum and an alpha lipoic eye therapy product containing DMAE, and recommended that she mix them together before applying them. The DMAE in the alpha lipoic eye product caused the loose skin to firm up by toning the muscles under-neath and eliminated the under-eye bags. The vitamin C serum thick-ened the delicate skin around the eye and greatly reduced the crow's-feet and crosshatched lines beneath her eyes.

The Proof in the Mirror

As Lauren started using ALA-enriched products, she quickly saw the changes in her skin. Within a few days, she noticed a decrease in under-eye circles and puffiness. ALA also reduced swelling in other areas of Lauren's face. The anti-inflammatory effects reduced the redness that was such a persistent and recalcitrant aspect of the rosacea. Within a week, a healthy glow returned to her skin. This was not an illusion or wishful thinking on her part. ALA's capacity to regulate production of nitric oxide, which controls blood flow to the skin, transformed her complex-ion from dull, pasty, and pale to vibrant and glowing.

Lauren's is a very happy success story. Thanks to the extraordinary anti-inflammatory properties of ALA, we were able to treat two condi-tions that appear to be polar opposites—the red, irritated skin of rosacea and the dull, lifeless skin caused by too little sleep, too much mental and physical stress, and elevated blood sugar from high-glycemic carbohy-drates, fruits, and vegetables.

Alpha Lipoic Acid

Characteristics

Powerful antioxidant, soluble in both water and fat. Alpha lipoic acid is called the "universal antioxidant" because of its dual solubility. ALA is also called the "metabolic antioxidant" because it plays a vital role in the energy production of the cells.

Function

· Gentle yet powerful—one hundred times more potent and antioxidant than vitamin C or E
· Promotes optimum efficiency for production of energy and aids in exfoliation

Benefits

· Able to reach and protect both water and lipid portions of skin with potent antioxidant benefits
· Protects levels of other antioxidants, like vitamin C and E, from depletion and works to increase their levels
· Dual solubility enables ALA to be available rapidly to the skin
· Skin develops a healthy youthful glowing appearance when treated with ALA

After several months, Lauren reported that her large pores seemed smaller and her skin's appearance was smoother. Just why this happens is not completely clear. Alpha lipoic acid can increase energy levels in the cell. Oil glands that are energy deficient produce abnormal ratios of oils secreted on the surface of the skin. When the proportion of these oils is off, the pores begin to clog. My theory is that alpha lipoic acid increases energy production in the oil glands, normalizing the oils secreted, which shrinks the pore size. Without abnormal amounts of oil clogging and stretching the pores, these tiny openings gradually normalize until they are invisible to the eye.

In my office practice, I have also seen ALA reduce the severity of facial scars by 70 to 80 percent. Studies have shown that alpha lipoic acid can prevent and reverse scar formation. A recent double-blind placebo-controlled study conducted by Dr. David Genecov of the International Craniofacial Institute and his group in Dallas applied alpha lipoic acid twice daily to the scars of cleft palate surgery on the upper lips of children. The parents applied the cream twice daily, not knowing whether the cream contained alpha lipoic acid. After one year, the study showed that the subjects who had received the ALA cream had much diminished scar formation—in fact, their lips appeared almost normal. The scars remained in those subjects who had received the placebo cream. In the future, alpha lipoic acid will be considered a standard treatment to help prevent and treat scar tissue.

ALA is particularly important for its ability to prevent the activation of transcription factor NF-kB that leads to the production of the inflammatory, toxic proteins called cytokines. There are no good food sources of ALA, so we need to take it as a supplement. In addition to ingesting daily supplements, I recommend daily application of ALA to the skin. I have formulated ALA into lotions for the face, body, and the eye area, and have used it successfully in treatment creams. You can find ALA available now in a wide range of creams and lotions.

I have my patients use ALA eye and face products in the morning under their moisturizer and makeup. It provides protection from the daily assault of free radicals on our skin and prevents development of further inflammatory problems. Combined with vitamin C ester at night, I have seen a marked reduction in lines and wrinkles; improved skin color; and reduction of dark, puffy under-eye circles.

DMAE

I first met Jenna in the green room of a popular talk show. She was a senior producer with all the high pressure and long hours her job entailed. Although only forty-two, Jenna confided to me that she was seriously considering plastic surgery. She had very few wrinkles, but her skin tone was poor, making her look a decade older than she was. Her jawline had softened and blurred, and the corners of her mouth turned down. Her upper eyelids and brow had drooped, giving her eyes a tired, hooded look.

One look at the food displayed for the guests told me a large part of the story. A host of sugary treats, ranging from Danish to doughnuts sat side by side with little boxes of cereal. A fruit bowl filled with bananas, apples, and oranges, and large pitchers of fresh juice completed the picture. The only protein in sight was in the milk offered as an accompaniment to the cereal or coffee. The choices offered provided nothing to repair the cells and plenty of foods proven to accelerate aging.

Jenna was bone thin—there was not an ounce of fat on her—another reason she looked older. A certain amount of fat is what makes our skin look plump and youthful. You may have noticed that people who carry a little extra weight, whether male or female, often have youthful-looking skin. I don't advocate overeating, but I do recommend you have enough fat in your diet to keep from getting too lean. Jenna's diet was lacking in quality fats and protein—a diagnosis I can make for women everywhere.

The loss of skin tone that was so visible on Jenna's face occurs as we grow older. The sagging is due in part to the decline of neurotransmitters like acetylcholine that stimulate muscle contraction. As we age, our muscles have less baseline contraction, causing them to elongate, to get loose and stretched out. This loss of tone results in sagging skin. Studies have shown that DMAE in salmon is a precursor to acetylcholine and can raise natural levels of this important neural chemical. In cosmetic surgery, the surgeon actually shortens the muscle by pulling it back and suturing it—giving the face a tightened, toned look. My goal was to find a way to eliminate the need for surgery or delay it for as long as possible for my patients.

You can see the effects of additional DMAE in the diet after eating all that salmon in the Three-Day Nutritional Face-lift. When DMAE is applied to the skin, the effects are almost instantaneous. The skin looks firmer, less lined, and smoother. If a pea-sized drop of DMAE lotion is spread on one side of the face, gently rubbed into the nasolabial fold, around the eye, forehead, under the chin, and on the neck, results can be seen in about twenty minutes. The side of the face with the DMAE will appear more contoured, the eye will be wider open, the nasolabial fold lessened. The effect is dramatic. There will also be an immediate reduction in lines and wrinkles. DMAE is also outstanding for tightening the dimpled skin on the back of the thighs and the upper arms.

I have formulated a product that contains DMAE and alpha lipoic acid, and have also added DMAE to vitamin C ester products. To ensure that DMAE is in your skin care regimen, look at the label to make sure it says "with NTP complex."

The short-term changes achieved from a DMAE-rich lotion will last eighteen to twenty-four hours. In the long term, the benefits of DMAE will be cumulative; your skin quality will continue to improve the longer you use the product.

After I left the talk show, I sent my DMAE products to Jenna with instructions to apply morning and evening. I also got her started on a diet rich in salmon. Finally, I reminded Jenna that she needed to drink eight to ten glasses of pure spring water per day. This would help flush toxins from her body and thoroughly hydrate her skin.

NTP Complex (DMAE)

Function
· Increases the appearance of toned skin
· Provides a healthy supply of nutrients that assist in the production of neurotransmitters
· Helps to maintain tone and firmness to face and neck

Characteristics
· Helps ensure adequate levels of neurotransmitters, which contribute to muscle tone maintenance
· Enhances access of vitamin C ester and alpha lipoic acid to skin
· Some may feel a tingling sensation as NTP complex begins to work, but NTP complex is still working even if no sensation is felt

> Benefits
> · Face, eye area, neck appear firmer
> · The appearance of lines and wrinkles are temporarily minimized
> · Immediate improvements remain visible for at least twelve hours
> · Benefits are extended by repeated use and sustained through use of day and evening treatment products

I have been told that a number of makeup artists now use DMAE under the makeup of well-known television personalities to create a firmer, smoother on-camera look. Even if you are not going in front of a camera, I recommend you use DMAE in the morning to firm and tone the skin for the day. Don't forget to apply DMAE body lotion all over to give a firm and toned appearance. This nutrient compound has powerful antioxidant-like properties of its own. Applied to the skin, DMAE is easily absorbed and helps to stabilize the cell membrane by promoting cell waste removal and by helping the cells absorb essential nutrients.

Jenna noticed a change in her skin within half an hour after applying the DMAE lotion. It was visibly firmer and the anti-inflammatory properties evened out her skin tone and color. After several months of use, Jenna's entire appearance was changed. Her eyes were wider, her brows lifted, and definition was returning to her cheekbones and jawline. She was eating salmon at least four times a week. The DMAE, fatty acids, and all-important protein were working to plump and tone the skin, rebuild collagen, and repair cellular damage.

Polyenylphosphatidyl Choline (PPC)

Since my business is concerned with beauty as well as health, I number many media personalities, models, and celebrities among my patients. They have to look great at all times—a strain for the rest of us even on our best days. These demands keep me searching for that next antiaging miracle. I know I've found it: polyenylphosphatidyl choline, PPC for short.

My discovery of this transformative food for the skin was motivated in part by a patient named Marika. A fashion model by trade, Marika was gifted with Titian hair and the milk-white complexion that often accompanies it—very similar to Nicole Kidman's coloring. Marika carefully avoided the sun and could put almost nothing on her sensitive skin in the way of treatments without causing an irritated reaction. No matter how hypoallergenic the product claimed to be, her skin reacted. The life of a top fashion model involves extensive travel, including frequent trips to Milan, Paris, London, and photo shoots all over the world. As anyone who flies often knows, the hours spent in an airplane dehydrate the skin. The bright lights and heavy makeup added insult to injury. Although she was only twenty-eight, her skin was already thinning and losing elasticity. I needed a targeted substance to get into the cell plasma membrane and actually help to rebuild it. I felt a responsibility to protect Marika's unique beauty and prolong her career for as long as possible.

My research led to the discovery of PPC, which offers protection to the cell membrane. Found naturally in lecithin, PPC contains nutrients that offer a wide range of benefits, including enhanced liver function and increased brain activity.

Polyenylphosphatidyl choline, or unsaturated phosphatidyl choline, is extremely important for the cell plasma membrane. The term "polyenyl" means there are multiple areas on the phospholipid molecule that have double bonds. The unique structure surrounding the double bonds provides antioxidant activity. When a molecule has double bonds it is called unsaturated, and this particular type of molecule can rapidly penetrate the skin, allowing its natural emollient characteristics to soften dry skin while acting as a powerful anti-inflammatory.

Bear in mind that the chief moisturizing agents in skin are phospholipids. When we apply an unsaturated phospholipid, like PPC, the moisturizing action is more effective and powerful than that of the natural phospholipids we find in our skin. PPC rapidly penetrates the cell plasma membrane where, thanks to its antioxidant capability, it can replace a fragile phospholipid. Every time one of these molecules is attacked by a free radical, an automatic defense comes into play. PPC stabilizes the cell membrane and delivers antioxidant action within its structure. At the same time, it provides tremendous emollient benefits to our skin to help heal dry, chapped, and inflamed skin, and it works against the inflammation that causes aging.

Polyenylphosphatidyl Choline (PPC)

Function
- Natural emollient
- Powerful anti-inflammatory
- Replaces phospholipids with self-repairing molecules
- Enhances delivery of other compounds

Characteristics
- Double bonds on molecule provide antioxidant capability
- Unsaturated; can rapidly penetrate skin and cell plasma membrane

Benefits
- Enhances liver function when taken orally
- Increases cognitive function when taken orally
- Helps heal dry, chapped, inflamed skin when applied topically

When applied topically, PPC is absorbed rapidly, offering anti-inflammatory, antioxidant relief to the skin—the results are nothing short of extraordinary. Since it is absorbed so quickly, it enhances penetration of other compounds used on the skin. By using the unsaturated PPC over your vitamin C ester or alpha lipoic acid lotions containing DMAE, you will enhance the delivery of these compounds into the skin, greatly increasing their efficacy.

PPC is a natural moisturizer. When applied to the face, PPC products produce a wonderful rosy glow. Patients tell me that after using PPC their skin looks as good as it did when they were children. You can see the emollient properties of PPC when used on winter-dry skin. Hands and feet, in particular, become dry and cracked in the low humidity of cold, windy weather. PPC reduces fissures and flaking in a matter of days. I have seen countless cases of hand and foot dermatitis characterized by drying, cracking, bleeding skin. The mainstay of dermatological treatment had been topical cortisone, which only works temporarily and tends to thin the skin. It is rewarding for me to be able to treat hand and foot dermatitis as well as severe dry skin with a natural ingredient like PPC and see long-lasting results. And I can avoid using powerful steroids on the skin.

Marika began to use the PPC every morning and evening. In the morning, she applied it over the DMAE/alpha lipoic acid lotion. In the evening, she applied it over a highly concentrated vitamin C ester cream. Within two weeks, Marika's skin had greatly improved. PPC not only helped to repair the lipid bilayer but also imparted gentle emolliency to Marika's face, which now had a fresh and youthful, rosy glow. All signs of dryness were gone. The DMAE had visibly toned and firmed her jawline and cheek contours. The overall effects were stunning.

Putting DMAE to the Test

Johnson & Johnson conducted an eight-week clinical evaluation of the effects of DMAE for skin firming and lifting. They tested fifty-three women, who ranged in age from thirty-seven to sixty, asking the women to use topicals daily for two months. One half of the group was given topicals with DMAE; the other half a non-DMAE placebo. The test was double-blind; neither the subjects nor those administering the tests knew which subjects were using DMAE-enhanced products.

At the eight-week mark, Johnson & Johnson evaluated the subjects' faces for signs of improvement in lift and firmness. As you can see in the following graph, the results were unquestionable. Those subjects who used topicals with DMAE showed significantly more improvement than those who used the placebo. They were evaluated on the basis of the depth of wrinkles around the eye, the smoothness of the cheek, a lift of the skin, and under-eye firming.

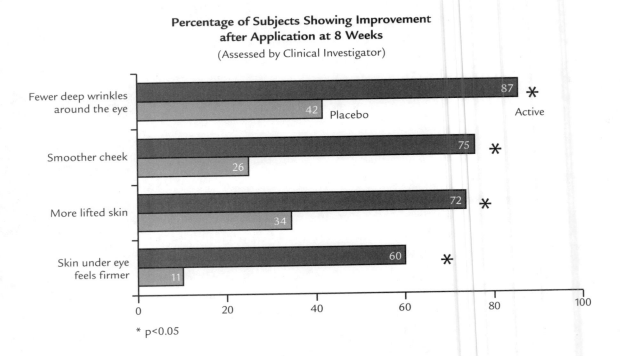

Percentage of Subjects Showing Improvement after Application at 8 Weeks
(Assessed by Clinical Investigator)

* $p < 0.05$

Tocotrienols—Super Vitamin E

The fat-soluble nutrient vitamin E is revered for its ability to reduce risks of coronary heart diseases and breast cancer and reverse signs of aging. A powerful antioxidant and moisturizer, it is just now becoming available in skin and hair products.

Vitamin E is made up of eight different compounds that are divided into two separate categories: tocopherols, the form traditionally used in beauty care products, and tocotrienols, the new "super" form, which is proving significantly stronger as an antioxidant. When scientists first studied vitamin E, they concluded that the alpha tocopherol was the most effective form of vitamin E for protecting lipid from damage by free radicals. This form of vitamin E quickly found its way into literally hundreds of beauty care products. Derivatives of alpha tocopherol, including tocopherol acetate and tocopherol succinate, were equally popular. Then, in the late 1980s, researchers began to look at other vitamin E compounds to see what effects they might have on health. They discovered that the tocotrienols reduced the risk of heart disease by slowing the body's ability to make cholesterol.

When I read about these discoveries, I wondered if tocotrienols had greater antioxidant potential than tocopherols when used on the skin. I devised a test to measure the effect tocotrienols would have on the cell plasma membrane. I found that under laboratory conditions tocotrienols are forty to sixty times more effective in preventing free radical damage than the traditional tocopherols. These super-E components are able to disperse rapidly through the cell plasma membrane and disarm the free radicals far more quickly than the tocopherols. In addition, I have found that tocotrienol-enriched preparations make hair shinier, reduce redness and flaking in severely dry skin, and prevent nails from cracking.

Tocotrienol

Function
· Powerful antioxidant and emollient

Characteristics
· Forty to sixty times more effective in preventing free radical damage to the skin than traditional vitamin E (alpha tocopherol)
· Fast-acting

Benefits
· Makes hair shinier
· Reduces skin redness and flaking
· Prevents nails from cracking

Holly provided me with the ideal opportunity to put the new to-cotrienol formulation to the test. Holly is African American. Her rich coffee-colored skin was firm, well-toned, and virtually wrinkle free. She had always enjoyed great skin. She did not make her first visit to a dermatologist until she was thirty-eight years old, when she came to see me.

Holly is a highly successful artist and set designer for films and Broadway shows. She works in a wide variety of media and had lately begun to experience trouble with her hands and fingernails—probably the result of one of the solvents or other chemicals she frequently used. Her nails were dry and splitting; the skin on the back of her hands was extremely dry and cracked, creating a painful and unsightly condition. She had had this problem before, but never with such severity. Holly was hard at work on a major production and could not stay home until her hands healed. She needed help immediately.

I started her on a PPC cream formulation containing tocotrienol and instructed her to massage it into her nails and the backs of her hands as often as three times a day. I gave her a lotion containing alpha lipoic acid to be used on her face. Holly was subject to occasional breakouts that left small facial scars that seemed to take forever to disappear. These were not truly scars but what are known as postinflammatory activity hyperpigmentation. The alpha lipoic acid, with its powerful anti-inflammatory properties, can reduce the appearance of these hyperpigmented areas in a very short time, sometimes in just a few days.

Don't Forget Your Hands

Your hands speak volumes about you and your lifestyle. They probably suffer more abuse than any other part of your body in terms of exposure to the sun, chemicals from cleaning products, and all sorts of bacteria. A good hand cream rich in emollients is essential to prevent the years from showing in your hands. Following is a list of creams containing my technology that I recommend to my patients:

· Alpha Lipoic Acid Body Toning Lotion SPF 15 with NTP Complex

· Phosphatidyl-E with Tocotrienol Lipid Bi-Layer Repair Hand and Body

Three weeks later, I went to the opening night of the Broadway musical revival that Holly had been working on. She had invited me to a cast party after the show. As she reached out both hands to greet me, I was delighted to see that her hands and nails had completely healed in less than a month! She reported that the alpha lipoic acid had so dramatically evened out her skin tone and coloring that everyone she knew was begging her to reveal her secret.

Olive Oil as a Beauty Product

You have learned about the extraordinary benefits of including olive oil in your diet. Extra virgin olive oil has proven healing properties when taken internally. Since the time of ancient Rome, olive oil has been used as an emollient. In the Roman baths, olive oil was an integral part of health and beauty rituals. The Romans massaged olive oil into the skin and removed it with a curved bone spatula, called a strigil. Since the oil was never rinsed off, Romans are recorded to have had skin that was beautiful, thanks to olive oil's powerful antioxidant and anti-inflammatory properties.

The polyphenols that are found abundantly in olive oil are extremely efficient and multifaceted antioxidants. Polyphenols are exceptionally stable and protective. The most powerful member of the olive oil polyphenol group is hydroxytyrosol. Extremely rare, and effective in even small concentrations, this superantioxidant, anti-inflammatory has been proven to be effective in improving general health and appearance. When used topically, olive oil results in smoother, more radiant skin.

Olive oil is rich in oleic acid, which is a superemollient. The essential fatty acids present in olive oil nourish the skin and provide anti-inflammatory activity. I have developed a line of olive oil polyphenol formulas that are suitable for sensitive skin. These products are a very gentle means of age prevention. Able to fight free radical damage without irritation, they are an ideal therapy for sensitive skin.

I have created an entire line of skin care products with olive oil. There are also many available in good drug stores.

Putting Theory into Practice—Skin Care

On the Perricone Wrinkle-Free Program, the goal of skin care is to avoid inflammatory ingredients and techniques and to provide antioxidant and anti-inflammatory protection. This simple skin care regimen takes only minutes each day. I will suggest products that contain the ingredients necessary to fight inflammation. You can find acceptable products on the shelves of your drugstore or supermarket, or you can splurge in the cosmetics department of your favorite department store. The key is to study the ingredients carefully and to make sure the products contain the compounds I recommend for skin care.

Cleansing

Don't fall for the myth that the best way to wash the skin is to use just plain old water. Nor do I recommend cleansing only with products like cold cream, as it can leave an oily residue that will block pores and provoke breakouts. If you use eye makeup, you may want to remove it at the end of the day with cold cream or a gentle makeup remover to avoid raccoon eyes. Use a cotton pad or soft tissue to remove the makeup, then proceed to wash your face as I recommend.

Some soaps are too harsh to be used on the delicate skin of your face. I caution against using antibacterial bar soaps on the face. You should use liquid cleansers that are applied by hand, then rinsed off thoroughly with lukewarm water. If you prefer to use bar soap, please use only the mildest soap available to avoid drying or irritating your skin. This style of gentle yet thorough cleansing will remove stale oil, dirt, and dead dry cells without damaging or drying the skin.

Buying Guide—Liquid Cleansers and Cleansing Bars

LIQUID CLEANSERS

- Oil of Olay Beauty Cleanser (Procter & Gamble)
- Formula 405 Deep Action Cleanser (Bradley Pharmaceuticals)
- Instant Action Rinse-Off Cleanser (Estée Lauder)
- Clean & Clear Facial Cleansing Gel (Johnson & Johnson)
- Cetaphil Lotion (Galderma)
- Neutrogena Non-Drying Cleansing Lotion
- Alpha Lipoic Acid Nutritive Cleanser (N. V. Perricone Cosmeceuticals)
- Citrus Cleanser (N. V. Perricone Cosmeceuticals)

CLEANSING BARS

- Cetaphil (Galderma)
- Dove Beauty Bar (Unilever)
- Oil of Olay Bar (Procter & Gamble)
- Basis Sensitive Skin Bar
- Neutrogena Bar

To avoid irritation, stay away from scrubbing grains, abrasive pads, washcloths, toners, and astringents. These can disturb the skin and produce aging inflammation. Don't overwash. Cleansing twice a day—in the morning and before bedtime—will keep your skin fresh and comfortable.

Moisturize: The Way to Luxuriously Supple Skin

Just as your diet must include healthy oils and eight to ten glasses of water a day, so too you need to add moisture to your skin from the outside, where it is exposed to the elements and pollution. Here are a few recommendations.

FOR OILY SKIN

- Alpha-Hydroxy Oil-Free Lotion
- Prescriptives All You Need for Oily Skin (Estée Lauder)

FOR NORMAL TO DRY SKIN

- Neutrogena Healthy Skin Face Lotion
- Oil of Olay Daily UV Protectant Beauty Fluid (Procter & Gamble)
- Pen-Kera Lotion (B. F. Ascher)
- Eucerin Face Cream (Beiersdorf)
- Face Finishing Moisturizer with DMAE (N. V. Perricone, Cosmecueticals)

Wrinkle-Free Skin Care

MORNING

1. Wash with a gentle cleanser.
2. Apply cream containing DMAE in combination with either alpha lipoic acid or vitamin C ester. Begin by applying the product to the forehead, working down over the face and neck, and finish up behind the ears.
3. Smooth eye-care products into the skin above and below the eyes
4. Top with a thin layer of moisturizer or, ideally, PPC cream.
5. Apply sunscreen if your moisturizer does not contain it.
6. Wait a moment for everything to be absorbed, then apply makeup.
7. Gently rub cream into your hands.

BEDTIME

1. Remove eye makeup.
2. Wash your face with cleanser, then pat dry.
3. Apply eye-care products.
4. Smooth on vitamin C–enriched night cream.
5. Finish with a light moisturizer.
6. Apply cream to your hands.

After your shower in the morning or your bath in the evening, use a rich body lotion all over your body. Concentrate on your legs, feet, and elbows to ensure that your skin is smooth and soft. Use DMAE to tighten up any dimpled skin on the back of the thighs and upper arms.

Skin Types

Everyone is unique. Rather than simply dividing skin care into categories based on the traditional dry, normal, and oily skin types, I evaluate my patients in terms of their skin and hair coloration. This allows me to develop skin care programs based on their individual potential for irritation and inflammation.

Northern European Skin

The palest complexions, especially in people of Irish and Nordic descent, are far more susceptible to sun damage. The lack of melanin in their skin leads to early signs of photo aging. In fact, when exposed to sunlight, light-toned complexions experience much greater free radical development than that produced in darker skin.

The melanin in the skin acts as an umbrella that absorbs ultraviolet rays. After just five minutes in direct sunlight, free radicals are activated primarily in the cell plasma membrane, which releases arachidonic acid, and the damaging cascade begins. In lighter skin tones, the cascade and its consequences proceed rapidly, leading to early wrinkling and, occasionally, skin cancer.

The oil glands of people with pale skin may be less active, which has the positive effect of limiting acne breakouts and blemishes. Unfortunately, lack of moisture leads to inflammatory chronic dryness and greater free radical production. Although pale skin is more prone to oxidative stress from dehydration and sunlight, it is less likely to scar or develop patches of discoloration. This type of skin heals beautifully after cosmetic procedures such as face-lift, dermabrasion, or skin peel.

If you have pale skin, you should use cleansers for dry or sensitive skin. Your moisturizer should be rich in emollients. This type of skin needs a lifetime of protection from sun damage. A sunscreen with a SPF 15 should be applied over the moisturizer and under your makeup each day. Be sure to use sunblock on your neck, chest, and hands as well.

African-American Skin

I was fortunate to do my residency at the Ford Medical Center in Detroit where 80 to 90 percent of my patients were African American. My three-year residency gave me a unique opportunity to learn about the wide variety of skin types among this population, and my experience led me to question two widely held myths.

Many doctors believe that since African-American skin is thicker than Caucasian skin, it can withstand highly concentrated treatments. I have found that although the top layer of the skin may be more compact, this type of skin does not respond well to aggressive therapy. In fact, I have found an increased inflammatory response that results in dark patches from overaggressive treatment. To avoid this problem, I recommend gentle, nonirritating cleansers and skin care products.

The second myth that I challenged was that African-American skin is more resistant to drying because it is naturally richer in sebaceous oils. I have seen many patients develop ashy dryness when they used strong soaps and toners. To keep the skin soft yet clear, I prescribe mild liquid cleansers. Even if the skin seems oily, scrubbing grains and alcohol-based astringents will cause hyperinflammatory darkening of the skin.

Moisturizers for African-American skins should be chosen on an individual basis. I usually start off with the lightest, nongreasy formulations. If dryness persists, I move up to a simple but richer product. Though Retin-A can be too irritating, darker skins can respond beautifully to mild alpha-hydroxy acids.

My research with African-American patients has demonstrated that because their skin is so sensitive, they develop an exaggerated inflammatory response to injuries. This results in the breakdown of collagen and elastin, resulting in scarring. It is essential that inflammation be minimized before it can cause scarring to African-American skin.

If cared for correctly, your African-American skin can have a smooth, youthful glow that can last well past age seventy. Your melanin-rich skin offers wonderful protection from aging free-radical production. Over time, anti-inflammatory effects of DMAE, alpha lipoic acid, and vitamin C ester will reduce discoloration and scarring and normalize oil gland activity.

Mediterranean Skin

This olive-toned complexion is intriguing for a number of reasons. First, it evolved within a population that had a naturally anti-inflammatory diet—large amounts of fish, very limited amounts of red meat, lots of olive oil, and a constant supply of fresh fruits and vegetables as well as generous servings of cooked tomatoes that contain high levels of lycopene, a powerful antioxidant.

Mediterranean skin has a bit more pigment than lighter Northern European skin, and the pigment is slightly different. Possessing an olive rather than brown tone, this skin has more sun protection than Northern European skin but has less of an exaggerated hyperpigmentation response to inflammation than African-American skin. In addition, Mediterranean skin seems to have a lower tendency to scar formation than that seen in the darker skins. Mediterranean skin tends to be oilier, which means it avoids the oxidative stress inherent in dry skin. The oil, coupled with more melanin to provide protection from the sun, delays the appearance of lines, wrinkles, and sagging skin.

On the down side, the active oil glands can increase the incidence and degree of acne. Fortunately, Mediterranean skin can tolerate aggressive antiacne treatment without developing patches of discoloration.

If you have Mediterranean skin, you should use a liquid cleanser designed for oily skin. Alpha lipoic acid will do a wonderful job shrinking pores that may have become enlarged from overactive oil glands. You should use only oil-free products, including the treatment products that contain sunscreens, DMAE, and vitamin C ester. I also recommend a special eye product containing alpha lipoic acid, which greatly diminishes the dark under-eye circles that plague men and women with Mediterranean skin.

Asian Skin

Asian skin has more melanin than Northern European skin, but far less than African-American or Latino skins. This provides protection from accelerated photo aging. Asian skin is resistant to sunlight and is less at risk for hyperpigmentation seen in African-American skin. The skin has just about the right level of sebaceous gland activity. There is neither a problem with chronic dryness nor is there significant acne.

The melanin content yields a skin tone that lacks radiance. I don't believe this is due only to pigment but instead is another manifestation of low-grade inflammation. This inflammation leads to water retention and edema that causes eye puffiness. Whenever there is underlying puffiness around the Asian eye, it is exaggerated by the natural bone structure. Alpha lipoic acid applied topically will resolve eye puffiness and also help normalize the microcirculation of the skin, resulting in increased radiance.

I have recently tested a new skin brightener called alpha hydroxy tetronic acid. This employs a nonhydroquinone molecule that is not irritating and lightens and brightens skin within a few days of application. This is a new substance and may not be available for purchase until 2003.

The eye-area puffiness and yellow skin tones of Asian skin respond beautifully to topical applications of alpha lipoic acid. Although sun protection is not as critical a factor as in Northern European skin, a light moisturizer with a bit of sunscreen will be a value-added product.

Latino Skin

The rich caramel-colored skin tones of my Latino patients have both strengths and drawbacks. On the plus side, the natural brown pigment provides a wonderful umbrella of sun protection. The inflammatory response in this skin is not as exaggerated as that of African-American skin, but it is still a problem.

I have found that acne is a frequent complaint. The overactive oil glands result in enlarged pores, blackheads, and blemishes. You must wash the skin twice a day with a liquid cleanser formulated for oily skin. Antioxidants, like alpha lipoic acid, DMAE, and vitamin C esters in oil-free bases, will shrink pores and refine your skin texture. It is particularly important that you select moisturizers and sunscreens that are not greasy and oil free.

Antioxidant, anti-inflammatory skin care takes just a few minutes when you get up in the morning and when you go to sleep at night. In an era of such expensive, high-tech antiaging options as lasers and micropeels, this simple and affordable approach seems almost minimalist in its philosophy. The results of the Wrinkle-Free Skin Care Program are fast and dramatic.

There are so many skin care products available now that promise to reverse signs of aging. I cannot vouch for their active ingredients as I can for my line of Cosmeceuticals, but these products are among the best available in drug and department stores. (See Appendix B.)

· Purpose Alpha Hydroxy Moisturizer, Dual Treatment, Moisture Lotion, Gentle Cleansing Wash (Johnson & Johnson)
· Eucerin Q-10 Anti-Wrinkle Sensitive Skin Cream (Beiersdorf)
· Nivea Q-10 Wrinkle Control Face Crème
· NeoStrata AHA Skin Smoother
· Aqua Glycolic AHA products
· Complex 15 products (contain phospholipids), Therapeutic Moisturizing Face Cream, Therapeutic Moisturizing Lotion
· Wrinkle Control products Eye Cream and Night Cream
· RoC Retinol Actif Pur Day and RoC Retinol Actif Pur Night Anti-Wrinkle Treatment (Johnson & Johnson)
· Lubriderm poly hydroxy acid–containing Skin Renewal product line (Pfizer)
· Nutraderm Therapeutic Lotion 30 (Galderma)
· Resilience Lift products (Estée Lauder)
· La Mer products
· Clarins products
· La Prairie products
· Shiseido Brightener
· L'Oréal Vitamin E products
· Cabot Labs Vitamin E products
· Alpha Hydroxy Gentle Cleansing Wash, Dual Treatment

Many of my patients come to me as a last resort before a trip to the cosmetic surgeon. After a few months on my full program, they no longer feel the need for surgery. Ironically, after a few months of special attention to their skin, especially with products containing DMAE, friends or coworkers often assume my patients have had cosmetic surgery. The new radiance in their skin, the correction of sagging, and the sense of health and energy they report are proof positive of the value of the Perricone Wrinkle-Free Program.

6

Go for the Glow: The Antiaging Power of Exercise

"Help me, Dr. Perricone," Rose pleaded. "I'm only thirty-seven, but I feel like I'm one hundred. I have no get up and go. I think, in fact, I might have chronic fatigue syndrome." I've certainly heard those words from many of my patients many times. Nothing will contribute more to fatigue than poor nutrition combined with a sedentary lifestyle. As Rose began discussing a program for a total physical and mental rejuvenation, she admitted to being sadly out of shape. She had twenty-five pounds to lose and was ready to change her eating habits by starting the Wrinkle-Free Diet. She had the diet, the supplements, and the skin care products. All that was left was to incorporate the fourth and final part of the program into her daily life. If looking and feeling youthful was Rose's goal, she had to start a fitness program.

I needed to find a way to increase Rose's energy level to get her up and moving. After the first week on the Perricone Wrinkle-Free Diet and supplements, Rose felt physically recharged. In fact, after only one day of eating adequate high-quality protein and avoiding sugar and caffeine, she confessed that she felt less sluggish and actually began to feel peppy. Rose considered this a major milestone.

I put Rose on glutathione cream, because it has been connected to significant breakthroughs in raising energy levels in my patients. I had witnessed the improvement of more than one case of chronic fatigue syndrome—in some instances in as little as four days—thanks to this powerful rejuvenator. (Remember Warren, whose story I shared with you in Chapter Four?) In a matter of days, Rose was pumped up to work out.

Why Exercise Works

As you have no doubt heard hundreds of times, exercise is vital for your health. There are mountains of studies proving that exercise can take off pounds, reduce the incidence of heart disease, lower blood pressure, improve mood, solve sleep problems, and even cut risks of certain cancers.

As a dermatologist, my first concern is beautiful skin, and exercise will help you to achieve just that. Studies have indicated that exercise benefits the skin in much the same way it improves bone and muscle quality. Without regular activity bones become fragile and muscles atrophy. When the skin of athletes is examined under a microscope, the impact of their high fitness levels is clear. The skin is thicker and has more and healthier collagen.

Exercise of almost any kind has a powerful, positive, anti-inflammatory effect on all our cells. Expending energy through exercise leads to an increase in vitality, but sadly too many of us avoid exercise. Too many people consider exercise a chore—a time-consuming, painful, or rigorous process. This does not have to be the case. Simple exercise, such as a brisk walk each day, can make a tremendous difference in overall health and beauty. The benefits of exercise—the increased level of "feel good" endorphins, in particular—can be addictive. Exercise is a wonderful tension reliever, a boon to our stress-filled lives. All of the benefits realized from exercise contribute to a sense of well-being, a higher metabolism, and increased strength. Once you begin a regular exercise program, you won't know how you ever lived without it. There are three separate but related elements of physical fitness: cardiovascular, muscle strength, and flexibility. Each requires a different kind of exercise, and each should be included in a complete exercise program.

Cardiovascular health requires aerobic exercise, like walking, bicycling, roller-skating, swimming, or running. Cardiovascular exercise gets your blood pumping and raises your metabolism so that food is converted to energy more quickly and burned up.

Resistance exercise or weight training builds muscle and promotes *muscle strength*. The more muscle mass you have, the more energy you use, and that means more calories are burned up! Muscle tissue is more compact than fat; if you have more muscle than fat, you will have a leaner, better-toned appearance.

Flexibility is an extremely important component in any antiaging program. The ability to move well—to have a full range of movement—is the best protection against injury. Being flexible will keep you active well into old age—and that is the secret of youth.

With cardiovascular exercise, the heart rate increases and blood circulates more efficiently, allowing nutrients to be absorbed by the cell and waste carried away. Exercise increases oxygen utilization, and oxygen is the basis of all energy production. You know that energy is the ultimate youth factor. Young cells have high energy levels, while older cells are characterized by decreased energy levels. High energy levels allow the cells to repair themselves and to resist stresses. Exercise, even moderate exercise three times a week, can greatly enhance energy levels on a cellular level, where the effects of aging take place.

Your water intake will increase as you exercise, because you feel your thirst more keenly. Adequate hydration is crucial to exercise. Remember: all important biochemical reactions on a cellular level take place in the presence of water. I have found that my patients who exercise regularly drink much more water than those who do not; as a result, their cells are better hydrated. This decreases inflammation, contributing to a youthful and healthy appearance.

Resistance training—using light weights—is proven to have great benefits. This type of exercise increases strength and muscle mass, and that protects you from injury from even simple daily activities. Increased muscle mass means that blood sugar is metabolized more rapidly (muscle tissue is very active and burns up blood sugar). This keeps your sugar levels low, which prevents inflammation.

Resistance training can also increase bone density. Bone density can decrease significantly with age, particularly in postmenopausal women who are prone to develop osteoporosis. Take a look around: you will also see many hunched-over, frail-looking older men. Early bone loss can lead to fractures later, which can be debilitating or even deadly. How many of you have an elderly relative who has broken his or her hip? A simple program of resistance training with light weights can ensure a solid, healthy bone density our entire lives, no matter what our chronological age.

Flexibility exercises prevent your muscles from atrophying and keep you limber, supple, and lithe. Stretching before and after you work out will protect your muscles from injury and has an all-over relaxing effect.

Rose asked me how running, swimming, and weight training could reduce wrinkles and restore a youthful glow to her face. In order to answer this question adequately, we first must explore the concept of fitness and how it affects the entire body.

What Is Fitness?

If you ask five different people to define "fitness," you will probably end up with five different answers. When I ask my patients, the answers I get range from "feeling confident in a bikini" to "being able to bench press three hundred pounds." Although such factors might be characteristic of a fit body, they are not necessarily so. The bikini wearer could be anorexic, while the weight lifter could be pumped full of steroids. Fitness is actually a biological measurement of the body's ability to function at peak capacity.

We know that exercise increases the immune system's ability to prevent infection—and even cancer. Exercise can lower our percentage of body fat, preventing the dangers of obesity, including insulin resistance, diabetes, and heart disease. There is excellent evidence that regular cardiovascular exercise can decrease the chances of suffering from age-related memory loss and senility. Studies have shown that people who exercise on a regular basis do not have the loss of brain tissue typical of sedentary old people.

Regular exercise is a mood elevator, and this is an extremely important factor in determining the quality of our lives. Many studies have shown that exercise can be as effective as an antidepressant drug in regulating mood. Elderly people who exercise regularly (as little as taking a daily walk) have a much lower incidence of depression. Further, when we exercise, we perspire and many of the body's toxins are eliminated in sweat.

On a purely superficial level, people who exercise have better blood circulation to the skin, giving it a healthy glow, which adds to an attractive appearance. Better circulation in the skin also decreases the chances of wrinkling.

Young versus Old—The Incomparable Power of Growth Hormone

Growth hormone is the true "youth" hormone. It is anabolic; it builds muscles, increases the vitality of the body's organ systems, and decreases levels of the stress hormone cortisol. This is in direct contrast to cortisol, which is catabolic and breaks down the body, leading to loss of muscle and bone, and loss of brain cells. When growth hormone is released, many positive things happen in your body. Growth hormone increases your learning ability, and has a positive effect on your memory in general. Growth hormone tends to reduce body fat and increase lean muscle mass, which are probably the two biggest obsessions of men and women of all ages.

Growth hormone release increases bone density and maintains the health of all our vital organs, including the heart, lungs, and kidneys. As we age, our body's normal release of growth hormone declines. In fact, it drops dramatically the older we get. This decrease leads to muscle loss, increased body fat, poor memory, increased susceptibility to degenerative diseases, and a slowdown in the ability to learn new tasks (like programming a VCR or Palm Pilot). Young people, on the other hand, who are treated to a steady release of growth hormone, have awe-inspiring learning abilities—often mastering complicated tasks, new languages, and names of hundreds of sports stars with ease. In addition, they are bursting with energy and—providing they avoid a steady diet of fast food, video games, and TV viewing—have no excess body fat.

As growth hormone production diminishes, we adults have one rabbit in the hat: exercise. It has been shown that regular exercise can increase the secretion of growth hormone in the body despite our increase in years. When growth hormone is released steadily, skin thickens, imparting a more youthful appearance.

Exercise helps to regulate other essential hormones in your body, insulin for instance. By exercising regularly, you actually increase insulin sensitivity in your cells, thereby decreasing blood sugar, an excess of which leads to premature aging. Resistance training can also raise levels of sex hormones, positively affecting our mood, increasing muscle mass and energy levels. Even a minimum amount of exercise can make a major difference in our lives. In this chapter, I have included some exercise regimens that will not require a great deal of time or stamina yet will provide an enormous payoff.

A Healthy Heart and Lungs

A strong, slow, steady heartbeat is the foundation of a healthy body. A strong cardiovascular system is essential for the delivery of oxygen to the cells, the ability of the cells to use oxygen, and for the blood vessels to carry away cellular waste products. Without adequate oxygen, every organ in the body suffers. To improve oxygen delivery, you must build cardiovascular fitness by means of regular exercise.

The heart is a muscle that pumps blood throughout the body. As a muscle, it is made stronger by aerobic exercise, thus increasing its ability to deliver more oxygen. Any exercise that increases heart rate—such as walking, skipping, biking, even jumping rope—increases the heart's ability to supply more oxygen with less effort.

To increase aerobic capacity, it is necessary to work the heart a minimum of *twenty to thirty minutes three times a week.* I advised Rose to take a thirty-minute walk at least three days a week. I recommended that she walk as briskly as possible but not to jog or run; she should walk at a pace at which she was not too winded to carry on a conversation.

For many years, physical trainers believed that effective aerobic exercise had to be performed at near-optimum or optimum training rate, which is 60 to 80 percent of your maximum heart rate. To calculate this rate, subtract your age from 220, then calculate 60 percent and 80 percent of that figure. For example, if you are 40 years old, your maximum heart rate is 80 percent of 180, or 144; and the lower heart rate would be 60 percent, or 108. Consequently, you should exercise at your optimum rate—between 108 and 144 beats. To track your heart rate, trainers tell you to take your pulse for ten seconds while exercising, then multiply that by six to get the heart rate per minute.

That's a lot to keep track of, and I feel it is totally unnecessary for our purposes. My goal for Rose and all my antiaging patients is to exercise *to increase oxygen to the skin,* not train for the next triathlon. In my experience, regimented, intensive exercise programs create enough problems and stresses of their own. If the exercise is too demanding, many people either develop sports-related injuries, or abandon a program that is too time-consuming. Over exercising can trigger the release of cortisol—the stress hormone that accelerates aging. The key to an appropriate routine is regular activity that slowly and steadily builds aerobic strength. It is always better to have regular, moderate exercise than sporadic, sweat-drenched workouts.

Muscle Strength and Endurance

Muscle strength, the second measure of fitness, is the ability to lift a weight, while endurance is the ability to lift that weight quickly and repeatedly. Strength and endurance are clearly related. Both employ weight training to condition muscles. Strength is developed by means of progressive resistance training. Weights are used in normal body movements, like bending the arm at the elbow. The weights are sufficient to overload the muscles, forcing contraction at maximum capacity. The resistance, or weight, is increased as the muscles develop. Gains are made most quickly from heavy resistance and few repetitions. Muscles are then allowed to recuperate for forty-eight hours until the next training session. Each session calls for four to eight repetitions, which is equal to one set, for each muscle group.

Endurance is developed in a program of sit-ups and push-ups. The key is repetition, gradually increasing the number that can be done before exhaustion sets in. For example, when you first start out, you may be able to complete only five sit-ups. During the next month, you will gradually be able to increase this to fifteen sit-ups, expending the same effort it once took you to complete the first five!

The Link Between Weight Training and Beautiful Skin

Hoisting metal dumbbells may seem an odd way to firm your face, but you can't argue with success. Resistance training releases growth hormone, while increasing muscle mass. It also lowers stress, resulting in lower levels of catabolic, destructive cortisol. For the skin, this means increased cell growth and repair and restored collagen fibers. Stronger muscles increase the body's capacity to perform, whether it is moving, thinking, or metabolizing on a cellular level. When the cells can successfully metabolize food for energy and repair, they are better able to handle free radical development and the accompanying inflammation. I started Rose on a simple program using three-pound weights. As her strength grew and the exercises became easier for her, she switched to five-pound weights.

Flexibility Test

Lean over at the waist with your feet apart. Without bending your knees, touch your hands to your toes. If you can effortlessly brush your toes with your fingertips, you are already on your way to a firm, youthful body. If you can't, don't worry. After just fifteen days on the Perricone Wrinkle-Free Fitness Plan, you will find new flexibility in your joints and muscles. Ability to use muscles to their full range of movement depends on good flexibility. Ligaments and joints that stretch

WARNING

Do not start any exercise program that increases your heart rate unless you have consulted your physician or are already following an exercise regimen.

easily enhance the body's ability to take on all sorts of exercise without risk of injury. Who wants to be stiff and creaky? Staying flexible will keep you young.

How Fit Are You?

When I finish my "exercise pitch" to new patients, I can see they are ready to dash out to the nearest gym to sign up for a lifetime membership. This enthusiasm is terrific, but before starting, you need to determine your current level of fitness in order to design the best program for you. The most accurate method of evaluating fitness is measured in a laboratory setting and gauges the amount of oxygen that is consumed by an individual as he or she pedals a stationary bike or runs on a treadmill. This measurement is called the VO_2-Max and refers to the maximum volume of oxygen the body can take in and utilize during sixty seconds of intensive exercise. The higher the VO_2-Max, the higher the oxygen intake and the greater the fitness level. For example, the VO_2-Max of marathon runners has been shown to be double that found in people who rarely exercise.

The VO_2-Max test, while accurate, is expensive. For the price of a stopwatch and a nine-inch-high stool, you can calibrate your fitness level in the comfort of your own home. Called the "step test," this three-minute trial measures the body's ability to recover from exertion. The quicker the body returns to normal, the higher the fitness level. This easy, inexpensive test not only tests current fitness levels but also allows you to measure improvement as you continue a physical activity program. The step test is quite safe, but if you are over thirty-five, or have a history of heart problems, check with your doctor before doing it.

The Step Test
1. Take your resting pulse. (Count your pulse for ten seconds then multiply by six.)
2. Place a nine-inch-high step stool on a flat, level surface.
3. Step up with your right foot, then your left foot.
4. Step down with your right foot and follow with the left.

5. Complete this step-up step-down combination in five seconds.
6. Holding a stopwatch, step up and down for precisely three minutes.
7. Stop. Rest for thirty seconds.
8. Take your pulse again.
9. If your pulse goes up *just a few beats* over your resting pulse, you are at maximum fitness level in the program.
10. If your pulse rate rises *ten beats above* your resting rate, you are in good to average shape, at an intermediate level of fitness—with room for improvement. Start the fitness program at the lowest range and work up quickly to maximum levels.
11. Pulse rates that are elevated by *fifteen beats or more* indicate poor to fair fitness. These numbers indicate that you should start out slowly and gradually build up endurance. You can test yourself at any time during the program to see if your fitness has improved and if you are ready to intensify your workout.

The Wrinkle-Free Fitness Plan

Whatever your fitness level, a complete program is one that combines exercises for flexibility, cardiovascular health, strength, and endurance. Rose's pulse rate was about fifteen beats above her resting rate—which was not surprising since she was a confessed couch potato. On the Wrinkle-Free Fitness plan, Rose did twenty to thirty minutes of aerobic exercise on Mondays, Wednesdays, and Fridays. She chose walking, which requires no fancy equipment and has the benefit of fresh air. On Tuesdays, Thursdays, and Saturdays, Rose did weight training. Each exercise session began with a five-minute stretching warm-up and concluded with a five-minute cooldown.

Since Rose is an early riser, making exercise part of her morning routine was easy. She just had to set her alarm a bit earlier during the work week to start the day off with a few minutes of energy-boosting exercise. She worked out on an empty stomach before she was barely conscious, and her exercise was almost finished before she was fully awake.

As she continued to work out, she looked forward to waking up this way—feeling on top of the world.

Not everyone is a morning person. Some like to break up the day at work or at home with noontime exercise. If this appeals to you, hold off eating until after you exercise. Others prefer to do their exercise as a transition between work and home, or between a busy day and the evening. With exercise, they are able to release the tensions of the day and start the evening refreshed and energized.

When you exercise is up to you. It does seem to work best if you have a routine. You can mix it up. Maybe you always do aerobics in the morning and weight training in the evening—whatever works for you.

You have to make certain that daily exercise is part of your life, an activity for which you plan. No one needs to persuade you to brush your teeth. Though the lack of exercise has far more severe effects on our health and appearance, so many of us still resist making exercise a natural part of our lives. I have designed this program to be done in the comfort of your own home. If you find going to a gym stimulating, then do your workouts and aerobics there. All that matters is that you find a way to exercise that suits you.

Warming Up and Cooling Down

Warm-ups are necessary to send extra blood to the muscles and joints, so that they can be ready to take on the work of increased activity. Without warm-ups, the muscles are stiff. They can be easily strained and stretching will be uncomfortable—and that means pain. If you prepare your muscles for a workout, you will reduce the chance of injury and aches.

Cooling down is equally important, because you need to reduce your heart rate gradually. Abruptly dropping the heart rate from peak activity to inactivity may cause you to become light-headed, and can result in serious problems. Your muscles should be stretched again after working out so that they will relax.

Are you ready to move? Let's warm up those muscles.

Flexibility Combinations

A supple, limber body is able to move quickly and easily. There is a healthy supply of oxygen in the muscles and joints that promotes growth and repair. The Wrinkle-Free Fitness Program has six stretching and flexibility combinations that tone and condition the entire body. They should be done for your warm-up sessions before aerobic or weight training, and for your cooldown at the end of the thirty-minute exercise session.

Wear comfortable clothing that is not binding. Boxer shorts and a T-shirt, sweats, or leggings will do. A sports bra is a good idea if you are full figured. You can do these combinations barefoot or in running shoes. You might want to have an exercise mat to make the floor work more comfortable.

Be sure that each stretching movement is slow and gentle. Done properly, this movement creates a light tension in the muscles and joints, similar to what you experience during yoga exercises. Do not do the bouncing and lunging moves that were the staple of high school phys ed. Those forced movements can strain or even tear the muscles, creating unwanted inflammation.

The exercises appear in the sequence in which they should be performed during your daily program. These combinations will work all of your body's muscle groups. The stretching feels great—it gets all the kinks out.

Do not be tempted to skip the warm-up and cooldown. These moves take only minutes and will help you avoid muscle aches and pains.

Flexibility Combination 1

To strengthen leg muscles, lean against the wall and put your right foot forward. Keep your left foot flat and knee straight. Hold for ten seconds. Feel the stretch in the back of your left leg. Repeat with your left leg forward and your right leg stretched behind.

Repeat three times.

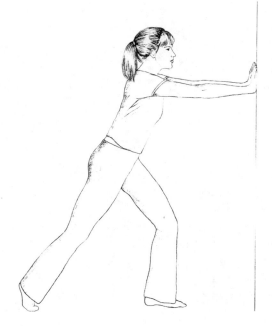

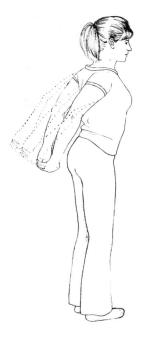

With arms extended behind your back, interlace your fingers and push your arms up and back. Keep your chest out and head erect. Feel the stretch in your shoulders.

Repeat three times.

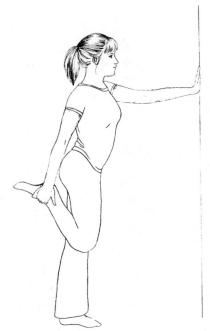

Flexibility Combination 2

Brace yourself against the wall and grasp one foot or ankle behind you. Gently pull toward buttocks with a straight back. Hold for twenty seconds. Feel the stretch in the front of your thigh. Repeat with other foot.

Repeat three times.

Standing with your feet together, place your hands behind your head and twist your upper body to the right, then left as far as you can go. Feel the stretch in your waist and lower back.

Repeat four to six times.

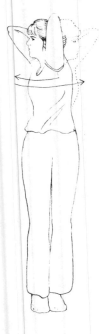

Flexibility Combination 3

Standing straight and tall, grasp the ends of a towel behind your head and hold for a count of ten. Feel the stretch in your shoulders and upper arms.

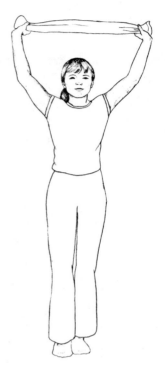

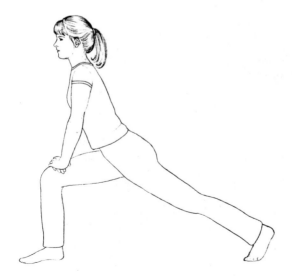

Take a large step forward with your right foot. Place your hands on your right knee and lean forward. Hold for a count of ten. Feel the stretch in both thighs. Switch legs and stretch on left knee.

Flexibility Combination 4

Stand upright with your legs just slightly apart. Stretch hands above your head, pushing them to the ceiling. Feel the stretch in your arms, shoulders, and spine. Hold for a count of five, then bend over and swing hands between the legs. Feel the stretch in the back of your thighs and lower back. Hold for a count of four.

Repeat three times.

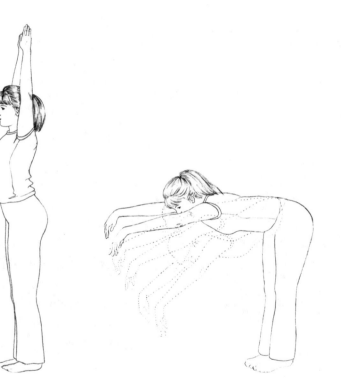
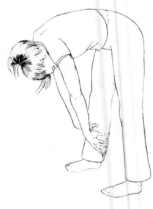

Lie flat on your back. Bend your knees and pull your legs to your chest with your arms. Hold for a count of six. Feel the stretch in your buttocks and stomach.

Repeat four to six times.

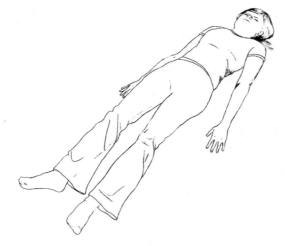

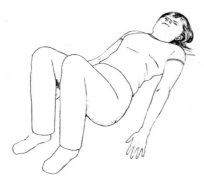

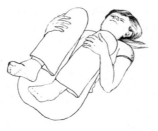

Flexibility Combination 5

Bend your elbows and raise your arms to your shoulders. Thrust your arms out to the side and back. Feel the stretch in your upper arms. Repeat four to six times.

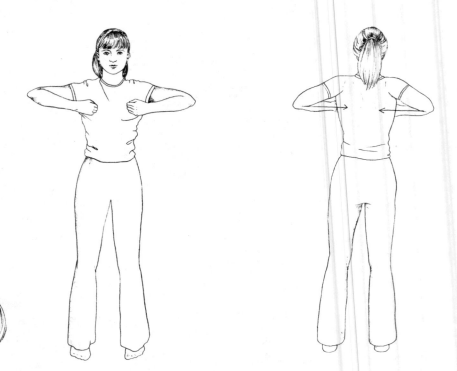

Raise your right leg in front of you with the knee bent until you can grasp your ankle or lower shin. Bend the knee of the standing leg if you have to. Hold for a count of five. Feel the stretch in your thigh. Repeat with your left leg.

Repeat four times.

Flexibility Combination 6

Stand straight with your feet spread apart comfortably. Clasp your hands above your head and lean to the right from the waist. Straighten up and bend to the left. Repeat and bend to the right. Feel the stretch in the backs of your thighs and your waist.

Repeat three to six times.

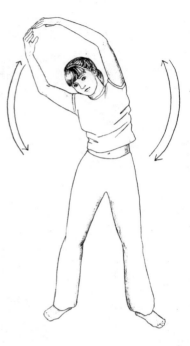

Lie on your back with both legs flat on the floor. Bend your right knee and pull it up toward your chest. Slide it back down and repeat the exercise with the left leg. Feel the stretch in your stomach and buttocks.

Repeat three to six times.

Remember, whatever type of exercise you choose, you must warm up and cool down before and after each twenty- to thirty-minute session. Start and end your cardiovascular or weight training exercise with a five-minute warm-up of gentle stretching. After your exercise, do your stretches slowly to cool down and gradually return heart rate to normal. Don't forget to drink a glass of cold water to restore fluids lost during exercise.

Aerobic Exercise

You need to accomplish a minimum of three twenty- to thirty-minute aerobic exercise sessions each week. This can include running, riding, swimming, biking, using a StairMaster, etc. If you are just starting a program, I recommend two forms of aerobics in particular: brisk walking and aerobic dancing. Walking is something everyone already knows how to do. You don't need special facilities or equipment. Even the busiest person can find time during the day for a twenty-minute walk. The pace must be brisk—no stopping for window-shopping or snacks. (I had one patient who claimed he gained weight on the program. It turned out that his morning walk took him past the doughnut shop, where he bought a different type each day and ate as he walked!) If you are already fit, you will need to walk farther and faster to gain physical benefits. Forty minutes of aerobics will turn your body into a fat-burning machine.

Six Ways to Add a Walk to Your Day

1. Park your car ten blocks from work.
2. If you take public transportation (bus, cab, or subway), get out ten blocks before your destination and walk the rest of the way.
3. Walk a dog for thirty minutes each day.
4. Take the stairs whenever possible.

5. In rainy weather, walk swiftly through an indoor mall for thirty minutes.
6. Park your car far from the entrance to the supermarket, mall, or movie theater.

The Dynamics of Walking

Walking works. That's what a study of out-of-shape middle-aged men and women showed when they walked on a treadmill four times a week for forty minutes. After five months, their VO_2-Max increased almost 30 percent, and their pulse rate dropped an average of ten points. Safe, simple, and effective, walking programs have up to half the dropout rate of other activities.

Equipment needs are minimal. Make sure you have a good pair of running or walking shoes that are flexible, light, and fit your feet well. Wear thick socks to cushion your feet. Special athletic socks designed for running offer extra padding and will protect your feet. In winter, a hat and gloves will keep you warm, since you lose most of the heat through the head and the hands. In hot, sunny weather, wear a baseball cap or a hat with a brim and sunscreen.

The correct posture and stance will deliver maximum benefits without provoking sore muscles. Stand tall and don't bend over or look at your feet. Try to take part of your walk uphill and swing your hands and arms naturally to increase the intensity of the workout. To burn more calories, try carrying one- to two-pound hand weights.

Dance Your Way to Aerobic Fitness

The other aerobic exercise my patients fit into and maintain easily in their lives is aerobic dance. It is not hard to find programs to join, either at an exercise studio, gym, or the local Y. In the morning, between the hours of seven and nine, you can usually find aerobic workouts on television. Click through the stations, and you will inevitably come upon an extremely fit man or woman leading an exercise class. Join in for twenty to thirty minutes and get a first-rate cardiovascular workout. If mornings are too hectic, buy some exercise videos and work out at your own convenience. The rhythmic exercise movements set to music are an excellent way to increase circulation and stimulate metabolism.

Be sure to keep the workout low impact. Jumping and twisting in aerobic exercise may increase the intensity, but it carries a high risk of injury. Studies report a 40 percent injury rate among participants and up to 75 percent of high-impact aerobics instructors sustain joint or muscle damage. Low-impact aerobics, while less strenuous, have a much better safety record yet still improve overall health and fitness.

Researchers have found that participants in a six-week program of aerobic exercise measured a 14 percent increase in cardiovascular fitness. Equipment needs are minimal. Wear a loose T-shirt and gym shorts to provide ventilation and freedom of movement. You can still wear a well-designed running shoe, but make sure that they fit securely. Wearing loose running shoes can quickly lead to blisters.

If this ends up becoming your favorite sport, you might want to look into shoes specially designed for aerobics. These shoes fit snugly with good support on the sides and have extra cushioning under the toe box. In aerobic dance, remember to keep your head up and your shoulders back. Bad posture will decrease cardiovascular impact and lead to back and knee pain.

Weight Training

Strength is built with weight training. Often known as progressive resistance training, weights (resistance) designed to tax the muscles are added to normal body movements. This forces the muscles to contract at a point close to the maximum effort. As muscles develop, the weight load is steadily increased.

Each time you lift a weight, the action is called a repetition, or rep. A weight-training program consists of a set of reps—a set being a series of repetitions for a specific muscle group. Most trainers recommend doing four to eight repetitions per set. Each set should be done no more than three times a day. It is important to take a brief break between sets. During the next thirty days, you will build up the number of reps you can do per set.

I have devised six weight-training combinations that work different muscle groups. When you do these exercises, move very deliberately. Do not rush. Stay in control of the movement. If you are just beginning weight training, use two-pound hand weights. You will need a pair of two-pound ankle weights as well. When you can do three sets of eight reps with ease, increase the weight you are using. As you get stronger, you will be converting fat to muscle mass, which is far more compact. You will achieve better definition. Women: do not worry about becoming too muscular. These exercises will make you lean.

> **Quick Tip:** Do not work the same muscles more than three days per week. They need time to heal and recover between workouts. Alternate daily with aerobics.

Keep cool water nearby as you work out. You can sip between sets.

Weight Training Exercise Combination 1

Stand straight with your arms at your sides, holding a dumbbell in each hand. Slowly bend the arms at the elbows and bring the weights up to your chest. Lower weights to your sides.

Beginner: do two to three sets of four reps. Work up to three sets of eight reps.

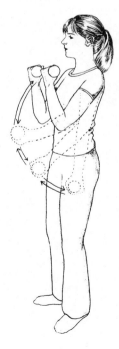

Lie on your back and hold a pair of dumbbells over your head, perpendicular to the floor. Slowly bend your right elbow and lower the dumbbell to your chest. Then repeat with your left arm. Alternate arms.

Beginner: do two to three sets of four reps. Work up to three sets of eight reps.

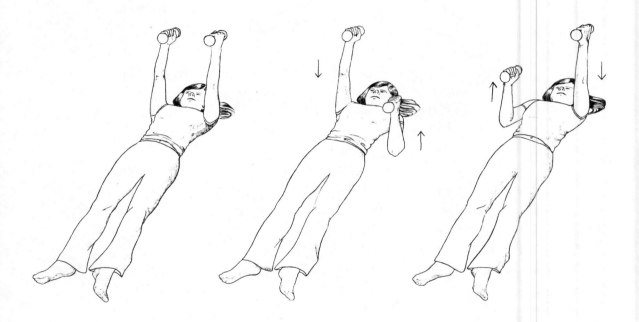

Weight Training Combination 2

Wearing two-pound ankle weights and holding on to the back of a chair, bend your right knee and slowly swing your leg back and up. Do reps on right side, then switch to left leg.

Beginner: do two to three sets for *each leg* of four reps. Work up to three sets for *each leg* of eight reps.

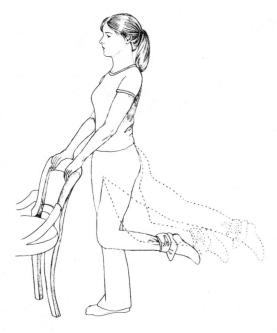

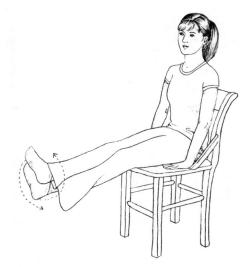

Wearing two-pound ankle weights, sit on a straight chair, stretch out your legs, cross them at the ankle, and hold for a count of four.

Beginner: do two to three sets of four reps. Work up to three sets of eight reps.

Weight Training Exercise 3

Lie down on the floor with your hands behind your head. Raise your head and shoulders until your shoulders leave the floor. Twist your body slightly to the left and lower body to the floor. Raise your head and shoulders again. Twist your body to the right and lower to the floor.

Beginner: do two to three sets of four reps. Work up to three sets of eight reps.

Note: In thirty days, you should be able to work up to three full sets.

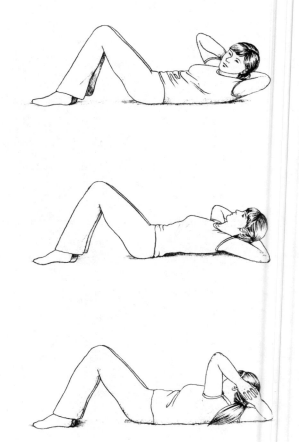

Weight Training Exercise Combination 4

Stand with your feet shoulder width apart with a dumbbell in each hand. Raise your hands to shoulder height. Raise your right arm to the ceiling, then down to your shoulder. Raise your left arm to the ceiling, then down to your shoulder.

Beginner: do two to three sets of four reps. Work up to three sets of eight reps.

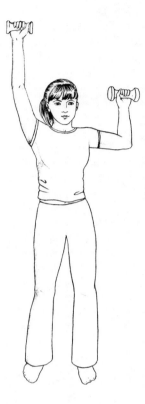

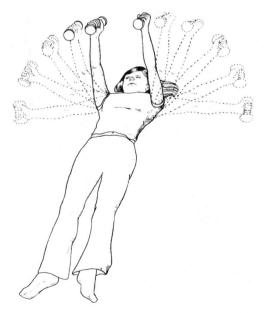

Lie flat on the floor and extend arms to hold dumbbells straight above your chest. Slowly swing your hands out and lower them to the floor. Bring hands up and repeat.

Beginner: do two sets of four reps. Work up to three sets of eight reps.

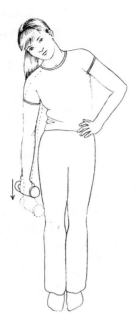

Weight Training Exercise Combination 5

Stand straight with your legs about twenty-four inches apart, a dumbbell in each hand. Lean to the left, bending at the waist as far as you can stretch. Straighten up. Do reps on this side. Then lean to your right side and do reps.

Beginner: do two to three sets on each side of four reps. Work up to three sets on each side of eight reps.

Lean over and rest your left hand on a chair seat. Holding a dumbbell in your right hand, lift your right hand to shoulder height, then lower your arm to straight position. Do reps on this side, then switch to the left side.

Beginner: do two to three sets on each side of four reps. Work up to three sets on each side of eight reps.

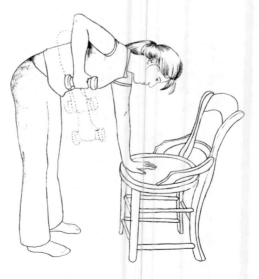

Weight Training Exercise Combination 6

Lie on your stomach with your legs together and your hands at your shoulders. With your knees and lower legs on the floor, raise your upper body until your arms are fully extended and your elbows straight. Lift your chin slightly.

Beginner: do two to three sets of two reps. Work up to three sets of ten reps.

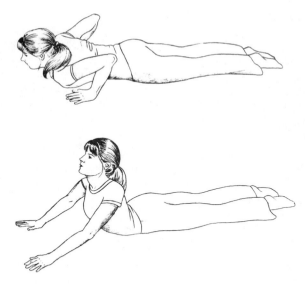

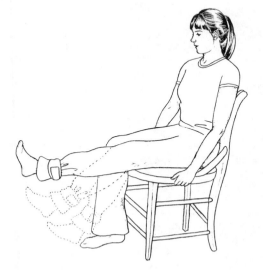

Sitting in a chair wearing ankle weights, raise your right foot until your knee is straight. Hold for a count of three, then slowly lower your foot to the ground. Do reps and then switch legs.

Beginner: do two to three sets with each leg of four reps. Work up to three sets with each leg of eight reps.

Remember, once you reach your goal, increase the weight with which you are working. That is the challenge of weight training: there is always room for improvement.

An Exercise Plan That Doesn't Quit

Even the best-designed exercise program will fail if it is too difficult and inconvenient to follow. The Wrinkle-Free Fitness Program is designed to fit real lifestyles. Most of my patients balance many demands—work, family, school, community. All these commitments require time and energy. My exercise program is created to be an automatic part of your day and a constant source of renewable energy. I am not training my patients to be professional athletes or even weekend warriors. Exercise is one aspect of the Wrinkle-Free Program. My goal is to provide an accessible, enjoyable program that does not have to overwhelm you. Work gradually to achieve your personal best. I want to increase your strength and improve your health by using exercise to reverse aging and inflammation.

The Wrinkle-Free Exercise Program

Monday
Warm-up: 5 minutes
Aerobics: 20 to 30 minutes
Cooldown: 5 minutes

Tuesday
Warm-up: 5 minutes
Weight training: 30 minutes
Cooldown: 5 minutes

Wednesday
Warm-up: 5 minutes
Aerobics: 20 to 30 minutes
Cooldown: 5 minutes

Thursday
Warm-up: 5 minutes
Weight training: 30 minutes
Cooldown: 5 minutes

Friday
Warm-up: 5 minutes
Aerobics: 20 to 30 minutes
Cooldown: 5 minutes

Saturday
Warm-up: 5 minutes
Weight training: 30 minutes
Cooldown: 5 minutes

7

Dr. Perricone's 28-Day Wrinkle-Free Program

Now you have all the information you need to commit to my 28-Day Program. You've learned about the nutrition, the supplements, the skin care, and the exercise you must incorporate into your daily life to rejuvenate your body and mind. And you understand the basic scientific reasons the various aspects of the program work. In this chapter you will find a day-by-day, easy-to-follow plan that consolidates all four aspects of the program.

After twenty-eight days on the Perricone Wrinkle-Free Program, you will see and feel the changes you have read about and seen in the photographs in this book. The success of my patients has demonstrated to me that this is a workable plan that is not overly challenging. Within a few days, you will have so much more energy that the Wrinkle-Free Program will become a way of life for you.

The Way We Live

The importance of your lifestyle is, of course, key in any general antiaging program. Your attitude and approach to daily life have everything to do with how you age.

The Death Hormone

Of all the destructive, proinflammatory and proaging forces I have observed as a physician, nothing compares to stress. Stress causes various hormonal changes in your body that rapidly alter cellular function in your vital organs. Not surprisingly, these effects are reflected in the appearance of your skin.

Since hormones are an important part of looking and feeling young and vital, we want to be sure to avoid anything that causes negative hormonal changes. In fact, as you age, all your hormone levels decline. There is a decline in sex hormones that give you your libido, muscle mass, and secondary sexual characteristics. There is a decline in growth hormone, as previously discussed, that plays a critical role in determining muscle mass, bone density, immune system health, skin thickness, and mental capacity. You may even see changes in the hormones produced by your thyroid gland that affect your metabolism.

Coffee and Cortisol

It has been shown that drinking just two cups of coffee can increase levels of the stress hormone cortisol. An elevation of this hormone can have adverse effects on the immune system, brain cells, sugar metabolism, and weight gain. In addition, coffee drinking has been reported to cause increased body fat. Although it is not clear why coffee affects weight gain, clinical studies show that by reducing coffee intake body fat goes down. When coffee drinkers substituted tea, especially green tea, they discovered that it had the opposite effect and helped them to lose weight.

Cortisol is one hormone that actually increases as we get older. We are all familiar with cortisol, because a derivative called cortisone is used in topical and systemic medications and has been part of the pharmacological arsenal for years. Cortisol is essential; it enables our internal systems to maintain stability and balance during acute forms of stress, such as fear, physical trauma, and extreme physical exertion. When it is needed during periods of stress, the body produces cortisol in the quantities necessary to combat that stress. However, a problem arises when cortisol is present for long periods of time and in excess quantities. When we measure the cortisol levels of a young person under stress, they rise rapidly, but within a few hours they decline to normal levels as the stress is relieved. However, when we measure cortisol levels in older people, the levels rise rapidly during stress but tend not to return to normal for days. Since cortisol levels continue to increase with age, a sixty-five-year-old person has far higher levels of cortisol circulating throughout his system than does a twenty-five-year-old.

It is toxic when large amounts of cortisol are circulating in our system for prolonged periods of time. Our brain cells, or neurons, are extremely sensitive to the effects of cortisol. When cortisol is circulating at a high level, it causes brain cells to die. That is why brain shrinkage is associated with senility in old age. Excessive amounts of cortisol can destroy the immune system, shrink the brain and other vital organs, decrease muscle mass, and cause thinning of the skin, which results in prominent blood vessels. In the antiaging field, cortisol is known as the death hormone because it is associated with old age and disease. When cortisol levels increase, blood sugar goes up with a resultant increase in insulin. This causes a burst of inflammation, increases fat storage, predisposes us to hypertension and accelerated aging.

Sleep: The Rejuvenation Hours

A good night's sleep can help you awake refreshed, looking radiant and youthful. And, after a good night's sleep, doesn't the world look better, too? A glance in the mirror shows that your face has fewer lines than usual. Eye area puffiness is decreased, and you have that certain glow that only comes with good health. Getting sufficient sleep is critical to the antiaging regimen, because, as you sleep, your cells undergo a process of repair. When we look at the hormone parameters during sleep, we find that sleep turns down the negative effects of cortisol and the "bad" neurotransmitters, like epinephrine and norepinephrine that can be elevated during stress. Growth hormone is released during sleep—and growth hormone is the youth hormone. A bad night's sleep results in high levels of cortisol, carbohydrate craving and weight gain!

A good night's sleep enhances cognitive ability. The day after a good night's sleep, you undoubtedly find that you think, problem-solve, and remember far better than you do after a sleepless night. During the sleep cycle, your body releases a hormone called melatonin that has positive effects on your skin and your immune system.

Since sleep is so important to the antiaging regimen, it is essential that we do whatever we can to enhance the sleep experience. A few alcoholic beverages in the evening may initially make us drowsy, but scientists know that after inducing initial drowsiness, alcohol precipitates a burst of norepinephrine in the system. Norepinephrine is one of the hormones that increases as a result of excitement or stress and is what causes many of us to wake up at three or four o'clock in the morning after drinking alcohol the previous evening. Hours after taking a drink, a burst of norepinephrine occurs that causes you to come back to consciousness. It is also important to avoid caffeine in the late afternoon and evening, because it, too, may interfere with your sleep patterns. In addition, before going to bed you should avoid any food that will cause a rapid rise in your blood sugar, as it will interfere with growth-hormone production, robbing you of this essential antiaging hormone.

I recommend that your presleep time be reserved for quiet and meditation. The bedroom should not be the place for important and/or emotional discussions with your significant other. This room should be your haven, reserved for rest and tranquility. Take this opportunity to empty your mind of all the details of your day—good and bad—or to pray, if that is your belief. In the daily plans that follow, meditation time will be indicated by an icon that looks like this:

I do not recommend the use of pharmacological agents to induce sleep, but one-half to one milligram of melatonin thirty minutes before bedtime is sometimes helpful in inducing sleep. Your daily exercise program will help, too. You will sleep more soundly if you exercise daily than you would if you are sedentary.

Before You Begin

Before beginning my anti-inflammatory, antiaging program, you have to stock up on the foods that are proven to take years off your face and body. These are the same foods that will improve your mood and keep your nervous system functioning at optimum levels. Many patients leave my office brimming with enthusiasm, carrying a handful of instruction sheets. On the next visit, they admit that they didn't follow the diet closely, because they didn't have the right foods in the house. That was the case with Emily.

When I first met Emily, she was fifteen pounds overweight. In addition to rejuvenating her skin she was hoping that she might lose some of her excess weight. With her fortieth birthday right around the corner, Emily was eager to get started. She had fine lines around her eyes and above her upper lip. She also had poor definition in her jawline, early signs of a double chin, and deep lines running from her nose to the sides of her mouth (the nasolabial folds). I knew how we could start changing her appearance for the better.

Once established on the nutritional and supplement program in conjunction with applications of lotions high in DMAE, Emily would be able to tone the muscles under the skin and dramatically smooth out the folds, restore angularity to her jaw and chin, and smooth out the lines above her upper lip. The program would also get rid of that burgeoning double chin.

I told Emily that if she followed the diet, substituted tea for coffee, and incorporated exercise into her daily routine, she would lose those fifteen pounds. Motivated, Emily made a vow to follow the diet and left my office with high hopes. But after a week Emily called in despair. She'd found herself coming home from work hungry, at which point she'd run to the fridge and munch on cold pizza or ice cream as she tried to figure out what she had on hand that would fit into the Wrinkle-Free Program. Obviously, she needed some help getting started.

As we sat in the office, I drew up a list for Emily and warned her that to be successful she first needed to put in a few hours of preparation and planning.

Phase I Preparation: The Food

To remove temptation and avoid falling into familiar dietary traps, I advised Emily to clean out her kitchen—to remove all the foods that were responsible for her extra pounds and wrinkled, sagging skin. I give you the same advice.

Emptying the Kitchen

Get several cardboard boxes and a few large garbage bags. Be prepared to toss out open packages and jars of proinflammatory foods. You can give unopened jars and boxes to your local charity food pantry. Start with the refrigerator. Gather up all the jams, jellies, and sugary condiments, as well as salty foods, like pickles, relish, cranberry sauce, chutneys, and syrups. Toss out bottles and cans of fruit juice and soft drinks. Now attack the freezer. Get rid of the packaged foods, even so-called diet or "healthy" meals, which can contain high-glycemic carbohydrates and transfats, as well as sodium. Knowing Emily's weakness, I told her not to forget the ice cream, cheesecake, cookie dough, and that extra pan of lasagna she kept on hand for emergencies. Stock your freezer with well-wrapped fresh fish. Salmon experts report that fresh frozen Alaskan salmon maintains excellent flavor for months.

What About My Family?

Some of my patients balk at emptying their cabinets and try to convince me that they need to keep ice cream and chips on hand for their spouses and children. This is not true. The foods that you are eliminating from your life are not healthy for any-

continued on next page

one. Children do need and should have dairy products and I do not believe in nonfat dairy products for anyone, especially children. Children should consume more healthy low-glycemic carbohydrates than I am recommending here for adults. However, cakes, cookies, ice cream, and soda are bad for children as well as adults. The most caring thing you can do for your family is to help them eat only the foods that will protect them from debilitating chronic illness. Even children are at risk for developing diabetes due to poor diets heavy in high-glycemic carbohydrates.

Next, throw out the trans fats. These include margarine, shortening, and peanut butters made with partially hydrogenated vegetable oil. Check labels carefully because many products contain hidden partially hydrogenated vegetable oils. The cheeses I recommend—and even these must be used in moderation—are the hard cheeses (such as Parmesan and Romano) and small amounts of feta used to flavor salads.

If you have any leftover fried chicken, Chinese food, luncheon meat, or bacon, toss that as well. Luncheon meats and bacon usually contain nitrates and other undesirable ingredients. You can find nitrate-free turkey bacon in the freezer section of your local health food store (and it's delicious, too!).

Next, work your way through your kitchen cabinets and pantry that are probably filled with at least six different half-eaten boxes of "healthy" cereals that are not healthy at all. Get rid of all cereals except old-fashioned slow-cooking oatmeal. Throw out the boxes of rice, bags of flour, sugar, pasta, instant mashed potatoes, crackers, breadcrumbs, cake mixes, gelatin desserts, and puddings. Move on to the breads, rolls, muffins, and pita bread—they all must go.

And don't forget the canned goods and the coffee, both regular and instant. Deviled ham, Vienna sausages, pastas, and sauces should all be tossed. Ditto the canned soups that are high in sodium and often contain a variety of unhealthy ingredients, including monosodium glutamate. Study canned soup labels carefully. Jars and cans of juice (except tomato and low-sodium V8), and all oils (except extra virgin olive oil) must go. Visit your health food store for healthy, low-sodium organic canned soups.

Last, but certainly not least, clean out the other sugars. In addition to white table sugar, this means brown sugar, confectioner's sugar, chocolate syrup, molasses, and honey. Although honey is a "natural" food, it is still pure sugar and will precipitate an inflammatory response. Take one last look for foods high in sugar, like drink mixes, hot chocolate, and flavored coffee as well as snack foods, including potato chips, pretzels, corn chips, rice cakes, and popcorn.

Restocking the Antiaging Kitchen

I tell my patients to shop in health food stores whenever possible. Though there are plenty of foods in the health food store that are proinflammatory, including a plethora of breads, grains, and chips, this is the best place to find organic produce and canned foods with fewer additives. Supermarkets are beginning to stock organic produce as well. If you buy canned goods anywhere, check the label for sugar and sodium content in particular. You can buy organic eggs laid by chickens that are fed a vegetarian diet high in the essential fatty acids. Though I cannot begin to list every available food, the following list will provide you with a good starting point.

I do not recommend that adults consume a lot of dairy products. However, plain yogurt and low-fat cottage cheese are quite acceptable. You can use a few tablespoons of low-fat milk in coffee and tea.

Recommended protein
- Skinless and boneless chicken breasts
- Turkey breast for roasting
- All of the fish listed on pages 56–57

A Word About Fish

Fish should be bought fresh, and it is always best to buy it the day you plan to eat it. Freezing can damage the flavor and texture of the fish. The intense cold ruptures the cells, giving fish an unpleasant, watery texture and stale flavor. Commercially frozen fish has given fish its bad reputation. If you think you do not like fish, it's possible that eating frozen filets has shaped your opinion. You'll find a world of difference in fresh seafood.

Of course, even fishermen freeze their catch. If you must freeze fish, the secret is to clean and dry the fish, double-wrap it first in plastic, then in foil, and store it in a freezer bag. That should protect the fish for up to a month.

Produce: Nature's Storehouse of Antioxidants

There are more than four hundred different anti-inflammatory bioflavonoids in a single serving of strawberries. Two stalks of broccoli provide more than 100 percent of the RDA for vitamin A. From asparagus to zucchini, fresh fruits and vegetables are a delicious and potent source of the antiaging antioxidants essential to health and longevity.

Recommended vegetables

- Arugula
- Asparagus
- Avocado
- Bean sprouts
- Bell peppers (green, orange, purple, red, and yellow)
- Broccoli and broccoli rabe
- Brussels sprouts
- Cauliflower
- Celery
- Cucumbers
- Eggplant

- Endive
- Escarole and other dark green leafy lettuces
- Garlic
- Ginger (fresh)
- Kale
- Mushrooms
- Onions
- Romaine lettuce
- Spinach
- Summer squash
- Tomatoes
- Zucchini

A steaming bowl of soup can be rich in antioxidants and nutrients. Water-soluble nutrients like vitamin C, calcium, and magnesium that can be lost in cooking are captured in every spoonful of soup. Keep in mind that soups that contain high-glycemic carbohydrates like pasta and potatoes are not permitted in the Wrinkle-Free Program. There are several soup recipes in Appendix A. If you do not have the time to prepare soup and freeze it in small portions, you can use canned soups, but be sure to read the labels to avoid sugar and too much salt.

Recommended fruits
- Apples
- Berries (blackberries, blueberries, raspberries, strawberries)
- Cantaloupe
- Citrus fruits (especially lemons for flavoring)
- Honeydew melon
- Peaches
- Pears
- Plums

Recommended beans and grains

- Barley (whole, for soups)
- Beans (including black, chickpeas, kidney, lentil, lima, navy, pinto, and soy—all great sources of fiber and protein)
- Oatmeal (old-fashioned, coarse ground)

Recommended canned goods

- *Alaskan* (wild) salmon packed in water
- Beans (black, chickpeas, kidney, lentil, lima, navy, pinto, and soy)
- Chicken broth (no-salt)
- Olives
- Sardines packed in olive oil
- Tuna packed in water

Recommended condiments

- Extra virgin olive oil
- Mustards (grainy and smooth—without honey)

Recommended frozen foods

- Flash-frozen vegetables with no additives (for emergencies only and can be used in soups and stir-fried dishes)

Recommended beverages

- Green tea (hot or iced)
- Spring water (buy big bottles to use at home and to refill smaller, portable bottles)

    Water is an extremely important component of the Perricone plan. Whenever water should be taken, you'll see this icon

Herbs and Spices

Herbs and spices provide wonderful boosts of flavor, but you need to read package labels carefully. Some, like garlic salt and onion salt, are

FOUR WEEKS
Johnson & Johnson Clinical Trial of DMAE

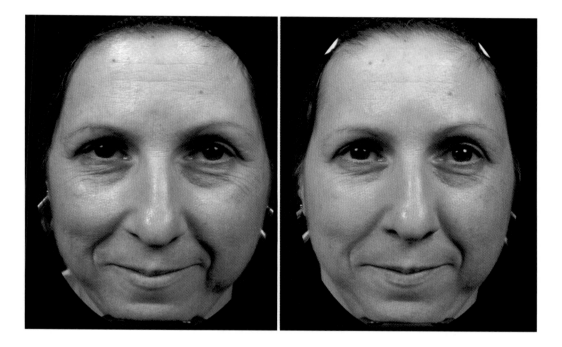

THE LINES ON THIS WOMAN'S FOREHEAD HAVE IMPROVED AND SO HAVE HER CROW'S-FEET. Look at the pores on her nose; they have shrunk noticeably. Her face looks thinner, her cheeks higher.

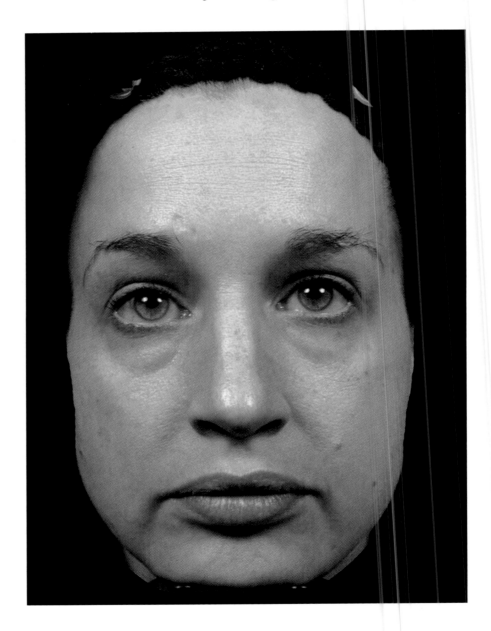

THIS WOMAN'S BROWS ARE HIGHER. SHE HAS LOST HER PALLOR.
The puffiness under her eyes has diminished.

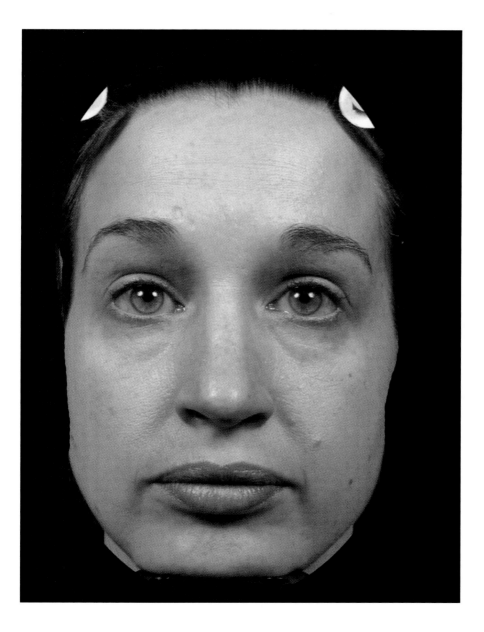

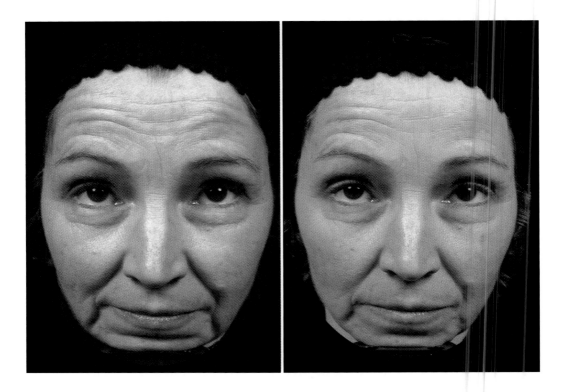

THIS IS AN EXTRAORDINARY IMPROVEMENT IN FOUR WEEKS. THE LINES ON THE FOREHEAD and between the brows are greatly diminished. The nasolabial folds are not as deep. Her skin tone is rosier.

for you to do aerobics and weight training. You don't want your workout to become a source of stress! Allow an additional five to ten minutes for warming up and cooling down. The type of exercise you should do each day is indicated in the program. You can work out at a different time each day—do whatever suits your schedule. For someone starting out, I find it is a good idea to pick a regular time to exercise so that it is part of your routine. Otherwise, it is easy to find that you're too busy to fit it in. If you set aside a time each day for these twenty-eight days, you will soon be looking and feeling so terrific you will look forward to your workout each day—it will become a time to de-stress and recharge.

Phase V Preparation: The Journal

Many of my patients find it helpful to keep a journal of their progress. You might want to record your reactions, feelings, and more tangible results—for example, your weight each day, the improving condition of your skin, and your increased energy. Whenever you feel tempted to stray from the program, pull out your journal and write down how you feel, whether a certain feeling or situation made you crave a food, want to skip exercise, or not bother to take your supplements. Becoming aware of the times, places, and feelings that induce you to stray from your goal will help you overcome temptation. Being able to see your progress will inspire you to stick with it. Your journal will be a record of how the 28-Day Wrinkle-Free Program has changed you and will encourage you to stay with it. There is nothing like measurable progress to keep you motivated to make the right choices for total beauty and health.

The 28-Day Wrinkle-Free Program

In the following pages you will find two weeks worth of daily plans, including menus, scheduled times for supplementation and skin care, and suggested exercise. When you have finished the first fourteen days, repeat the daily plans from the beginning to complete the full, four-week program. Some of the menus indicate a range of protein serving sizes (for example, from 3 to 6 ounces). If you are larger, have more muscle mass, and/or are physically active, you will use the higher amounts. For example, a lower amount of protein would be appropriate for a sedentary woman approximately 5'4" tall and weighing 130 pounds.

An asterisk next to a menu item indicates that the recipe can be found in Appendix A. The recipes I've included are easy, quick, and tasty and require a minimum of preparation. I've also included some delicious ways to prepare protein using some foolproof recipes for fish and chicken.

Protein First!

Always remember to eat the protein first at every meal. It may seem odd to eat your fish before your soup, but doing so will ensure that you will avoid a glycemic response.

Week One

Day 1: Monday
Exercise for the day: aerobics
Wake up

BREAKFAST
- 3 to 4 ounces smoked Nova Scotia salmon
- ½ cup slow-cooked oatmeal with 2 tablespoons blueberries
- 1 teaspoon slivered almonds
- Green tea or water

LUNCH
- 4- to 6-ounce broiled turkey burger (no bun)
- Lettuce and tomato
- ½ cup Three-Bean Salad★
- 1 cup water or green tea

AFTERNOON SNACK
- 2 ounces sliced turkey or chicken breast
- 4 hazelnuts
- 4 celery sticks

DINNER
- 4 to 6 ounces broiled salmon
- 1 cup lentil soup
- Tossed green salad dressed with olive oil and lemon juice
- ½ cup steamed spinach
- Cold water or green tea

BEDTIME SNACK
- 1 hard-boiled egg
- 3 celery sticks
- 3 red bell pepper strips
- 3 green olives

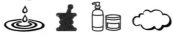

Day 2: Tuesday
Exercise for the day: weight training
Wake up

BREAKFAST
- Omelet made with 3 egg whites and one yolk
- Sliced tomato
- ½ cup blueberries
- Tea or water

LUNCH
- 3 to 6 ounces smoked or grilled salmon
- Green salad with tomatoes, cucumbers, onions and 2 tablespoons chickpeas dressed with olive oil, lemon juice, and garlic

AFTERNOON SNACK
- ½ cup low-fat cottage cheese
- 4 small black olives
- 4 endive spears

DINNER
- 4 to 6 ounces baked or grilled halibut
- 1 cup Chicken-Vegetable Soup★
- Salad of romaine lettuce, chopped avocado, tomato, green onion, and celery dressed with olive oil and lemon juice

BEDTIME SNACK
- 2 ounces sliced roast turkey breast
- 6 whole almonds
- 2-inch wedge of honeydew melon

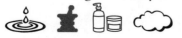

Day 3: Wednesday
Exercise for the day: aerobics
Wake up

BREAKFAST
- 2 slices turkey bacon
- 6 ounces plain yogurt
- ½ cup strawberries
- 3 hazelnuts
- Tea or water

LUNCH
- 3- to 4-ounce can water-packed tuna
- 1 cup sliced tomatoes and cucumbers
- ½ cup bean salad

AFTERNOON SNACK
- 2 ounces sliced turkey breast
- 4 almonds
- 1 small pear

DINNER
- 4 to 6 ounces broiled filet of salmon. (Make 8 ounces and save
  2 ounces for tomorrow's bedtime snack.)
- ¼ cup green beans

- Spinach salad with mushrooms, slice of red onion, and ¼ cup chickpeas, dressed with olive oil and lemon juice

BEDTIME SNACK
- 2 ounces Grilled Chicken Breast★
- ¼ cup raw cauliflower
- 4 black olives

Day 4: Thursday

Exercise for the day: weight training

Wake up

BREAKFAST
- 1 slice of Canadian bacon or 2 slices turkey bacon
- 2 poached egg whites and one yolk
- ½ cup cooked oatmeal
- ½ cup blueberries
- Green or black tea

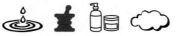

LUNCH
- 4 ounces grilled chicken salad (with fresh dill, chopped red onion, garlic, and olive oil)
- ½ cup steamed broccoli
- ½ cup strawberries
- Green tea or water

AFTERNOON SNACK
- 2 slices roast turkey breast
- 4 cherry tomatoes
- 4 almonds

DINNER
- 6 ounces broiled filet of sole, cod, or scrod. (Make 8 ounces and save two ounces for tomorrow's bedtime snack.)
- 8 Oven-Roasted Brussels Sprouts with Apples★
- Romaine lettuce salad with 2 ounces chickpeas, dressed with olive oil, garlic, and lemon juice

BEDTIME SNACK
- 2 ounces salmon
- 2 tablespoons Cuban Black Bean Salad★

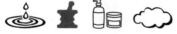

Day 5: Friday
Exercise for the day: aerobics
Wake up

BREAKFAST
- 4 ounces smoked salmon
- ½ cup slow-cooked oatmeal seasoned with cinnamon
- 2 teaspoons chopped almonds
- 2-inch wedge of cantaloupe
- Tea or water

LUNCH
- 4 ounces salmon salad (finely cubed salmon filet or canned salmon dressed with lemon juice, olive oil, and dill)
- A few leaves of Romaine lettuce
- ½ cup lentil soup
- Water or green tea

AFTERNOON SNACK
- 2 slices turkey
- ½ cup strawberries
- 4 hazelnuts

DINNER
- 1 roast chicken breast (skin removed)
- ½ cup grilled zucchini
- ½ cup Three Bean Salad★

BEDTIME SNACK
- 2 ounces cold filet of sole, cod, or scrod
- 3 macadamia nuts
- 3 cherry tomatoes

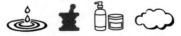

Day 6: Saturday
Exercise for the day: weight training
Wake up

BREAKFAST
- Omelet of 3 egg whites and 1 yolk with a few sliced mushrooms and a little spinach
- 1 slice Canadian or turkey bacon
- 2-inch wedge of honeydew melon
- Tea or water

LUNCH
- 4 to 6 ounces broiled salmon
- Caesar salad *without* croutons
- ½ apple

AFTERNOON SNACK
- 1 hard-boiled egg
- ½ cup sliced strawberries
- 3 almonds

DINNER
- 4 to 6 ounces grilled halibut
- Tossed Greek salad made with romaine lettuce, 3 black olives, 1 ounce feta cheese, ½ cucumber, 4 cherry tomatoes; dressed with olive oil, lemon juice, and a dash of oregano, mixed to taste
- Steamed or Grilled Asparagus★
- 2-inch wedge of cantaloupe

BEDTIME SNACK
- 2 slices roast turkey or chicken breast
- 4 macadamia nuts
- Small peach or nectarine

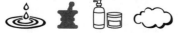

Day 7: Sunday
Exercise for the day: relaxation
Wake up

BREAKFAST
- 3 to 6 ounces broiled salmon
- ½ cup slow-cooked oatmeal
- 2-inch wedge of cantaloupe
- Tea or water

LUNCH
- Crabmeat salad made with a 6-ounce can of crabmeat, 1 chopped scallion, 1 chopped celery rib; dress with ¼ cup yogurt, juice of ½ lemon; serve inside ½ avocado
- 1 cup strawberries
- Water or green tea

AFTERNOON SNACK
- ½ cup cottage cheese
- 4 almonds
- 1 apple

DINNER
- Grilled chicken breast
- ¾ cup roasted or sautéed mushrooms and Sautéed Zucchini or Summer Squash★
- Romaine lettuce salad, sliced tomatoes, fresh basil with 1 ounce

grated Parmesan cheese, dressed with olive oil and lemon juice, mixed to taste
- ½ cup fresh berries

BEDTIME SNACK
- 2 slices of turkey breast
- 3 olives
- 1 pear

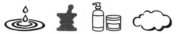

Week Two

Day 8: Monday
Exercise for the day: aerobics
Wake up

BREAKFAST
- 2 slices Canadian bacon, ham, or turkey bacon
- ½ cup low-fat cottage cheese
- ½ cup blueberries
- Tea or water

LUNCH
- 3- to 4-ounce can water-packed tuna
- ½ cup lentil soup
- Romaine lettuce salad topped with chopped tomato and red onion; dress with olive oil and lemon
- Tea

AFTERNOON SNACK
- 2 ounces smoked salmon
- 2-inch wedge cantaloupe

DINNER
- 6 ounces Scallops with Garlic and Parsley★ (cook 8 ounces and save 2 ounces for tomorrow's lunch)
- Mediterranean Chopped Salad★ with ½ cup chickpeas
- ½ cup cooked green beans
- Water or green tea

BEDTIME SNACK
- 2 slices turkey breast
- 4 green olives
- 1 apple

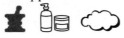

Day 9: Tuesday

Exercise for the day: weight training

Wake-up

BREAKFAST
- Egg white omelet made with 3 to 4 egg whites and one yolk (add a few sliced mushrooms, if desired)
- ½ cup oatmeal
- 3 hazelnuts
- Tea or water

LUNCH
- Scallop salad (2 ounces scallops from previous night's dinner); dress with olive oil, lemon juice, chopped red onion, and dill
- ½ cup Three Bean Salad★
- Water or green tea

AFTERNOON SNACK
- 2 ounces smoked salmon
- 4 black olives
- 3 endive spears

DINNER
- 6 ounces grilled salmon
- ½ cup Cuban Black Bean Soup★
- Romaine salad dressed with olive oil and lemon juice
- ½ cup berries
- Water or green tea

BEDTIME SNACK
- ½ cup cottage cheese
- ½ cup strawberries
- 4 macadamia nuts

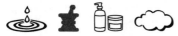

Day 10: Wednesday
Exercise for the day: aerobics
Wake up

BREAKFAST
- 2 slices turkey bacon
- 1 cup plain yogurt
- ½ cup strawberries
- 3 almonds
- Tea or water

LUNCH
- 4 to 6 ounces grilled chicken
- ½ cup vegetable barley soup
- Large green salad with sliced tomatoes
- 2-inch wedge of cantaloupe
- Water or green tea

AFTERNOON SNACK
- 1 hard-boiled egg
- 2-inch wedge of cantaloupe
- 4 almonds

DINNER
- 6 ounces broiled flounder filet
- Tricolor salad (arugula, radicchio, and endive) with ½ cup kidney beans or soybeans, dressed with olive oil and lemon juice
- Sautéed Spinach★
- Water or tea

BEDTIME SNACK
- 2 slices chicken or turkey breast
- 4 macadamia nuts
- 1 small peach

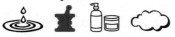

Day 11: Thursday
Exercise for the day: weight training
Wake up

BREAKFAST
- 4 ounces smoked salmon
- 3 ounces plain yogurt
- 1 tomato slice
- ¼ cantaloupe
- Tea or water

LUNCH
- 6-ounces canned crabmeat dressed with 1 tablespoon mayonnaise
- ½ cup lentil soup
- Large romaine lettuce salad dressed with olive oil and lemon to taste
- Water or green tea

AFTERNOON SNACK
- 1 hard-boiled egg
- 4 cherry tomatoes
- 4 macadamia nuts

DINNER
- 6 ounces roast chicken breast (cook 8 ounces and save 2 ounces for tomorrow's lunch)
- ½ cup Manhattan Clam Chowder★

- ½ cup grilled eggplant topped with sliced tomato and 1 tablespoon grated Parmesan cheese
- Water or green tea

BEDTIME SNACK
- ½ cup low-fat cottage cheese
- ½ cup blueberries
- 4 hazelnuts

Day 12: Friday
Exercise for the day: aerobics
Wake up

BREAKFAST
- Scrambled eggs (3 egg whites and 1 yolk) with a little chopped onion and green bell peppers
- 2 slices turkey bacon
- 2-inch wedge cantaloupe
- Tea or water

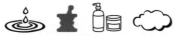

LUNCH
- 3 to 5 ounces of chicken salad (made with 2 ounces chicken saved from last night's dinner, mixed with chopped red onion and celery, and dressed with 1 tablespoon olive oil and lemon juice) served on a bed of romaine lettuce
- Sliced tomatoes
- 1 cup Chicken-Vegetable Soup★
- Water or green tea

AFTERNOON SNACK
- ½ cup plain yogurt
- ½ cup blueberries
- 1 teaspoon chopped almonds

DINNER
- 6 ounces grilled salmon
- Salad of romaine lettuce, avocado, and tomato, dressed with olive oil and lemon juice
- Grilled zucchini and mushroom kebobs
- Water or green tea

BEDTIME SNACK
- 2 ounces tuna salad (water-packed tuna mixed with onion, celery, pepper, and mustard or a touch of mayonnaise, if desired)
- 4 almonds
- 1 pear

Day 13: Saturday
Exercise for the day: aerobics
Wake up

BREAKFAST
- 2 to 4 ounces smoked salmon
- ½ cup plain yogurt
- 1 tablespoon chopped walnuts
- ½ cup blueberries
- Tea or water

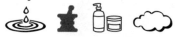

LUNCH
- Grilled Chicken Breast★
- Green salad topped with ½ cup white or navy beans
- Steamed asparagus
- Water or green tea

AFTERNOON SNACK
- 1 hard-boiled egg
- 2-inch wedge cantaloupe
- 4 macadamia nuts

DINNER
- 6 ounces grilled bluefin or albacore tuna steak
- ½ cup grilled zucchini, eggplant, and red or green bell pepper lightly drizzled with olive oil and sprinkled with 1 tablespoon Parmesan cheese
- Tomato salsa (use fresh, if possible)
- Water or green tea

BEDTIME SNACK
- 2 slices turkey breast
- 4 green olives
- 4 cherry tomatoes

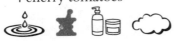

Day 14: Sunday
Exercise for the day: relaxation
Wake up

BREAKFAST
- Omelet made with 3 to 4 egg whites, 1 yolk, and a few sliced fresh mushrooms
- ½ cup slow-cooked oatmeal
- 1 teaspoon chopped almonds
- 2-inch wedge cantaloupe
- Tea or water

LUNCH
- 3 to 4 ounces water-packed tuna
- Romaine lettuce salad made with ½ cup white beans, ¼ cup crumbled feta cheese, 4 cherry tomatoes, and slice red onion, dressed with olive oil and lemon juice
- Water or green tea

AFTERNOON SNACK
- 1 slice turkey breast
- 4 hazelnuts
- 2-inch wedge cantaloupe

DINNER
- 4 large shrimp, grilled, broiled, or baked on skewers with mushrooms, onions, and cherry tomatoes
- ½ cup Cuban Black Bean Soup★
- Romaine lettuce salad dressed with olive oil and lemon juice
- Water or green tea

BEDTIME SNACK
- ½ cup low-fat cottage cheese
- 4 almonds
- ½ pear

Congratulations! Now that you have finished the first fourteen days of the Perricone Wrinkle-Free Program you should be feeling terrific, and your skin must be glowing. Most of my patients' journal entries are extremely upbeat at this point, and I'm sure yours will be, too. Now that the Wrinkle-Free Program has started to work its magic on you, you should have the confidence and enthusiasm to repeat the two weeks you have just finished to complete the 28-Day Program. And by the time you have done that, you will be well on your way to being wrinkle-free for life!

8

The Ageless Future: Developing Technologies

I began this book by considering how our lives are being extended by scientific breakthroughs in every field. I have discussed my own discoveries regarding inflammation and efforts to restore and preserve youthful skin. And I have designed my 28-Day Wrinkle-Free Program to bring total health and beauty to your life. It seems appropriate to conclude by looking forward to new technologies that are being developed to fight aging.

Cutting-edge research is currently being done on spin traps, light therapy, electrical and chemical stimulation of muscles, tetronic acid, telomerase, and thymic hormones and growth hormone releases. In addition I am continuing my research on new ways of delivering nutrients and medications to the body with transdermal delivery systems. We are on the brink of a whole new world of treatments to prevent aging. In the years to come, you will be reading about, hearing about, and using these revolutionary new technologies. I am confident that they will forever change how we age. Of course, I plan to continue making my own contributions to this exciting field.

Spin Traps

Spin traps are molecules that have been used as research tools to study free radicals. Since free radicals exist only for a nanosecond, it is very difficult to study these reactive molecules, whether in the test tube or the human body. Spin traps catch and hold free radicals. When bonded with a spin trap, a free radical's life is extended beyond its normal fraction of a second, allowing it to be measured and studied. But spin traps have proven to be much more than just research aids or diagnostic tools. They are extremely therapeutic.

When captured by spin traps, free radicals become inactivated, unable to do their normal damage. Once caught and disabled by the spin traps, the free radical is prevented from damaging the cell plasma membrane. As you know, that means spin traps are powerful anti-inflammatories.

Great progress has been made in the search for more powerful spin traps with low toxicity. Dr. David Becker of the University of Florida, has conducted research on several new spin traps, specifically those called nitrones. Dr. Becker has discovered a class of nitrones called azulenes. It is interesting that the azuleneyl nitrones turn color, from green to violet, when they capture free radicals. This means that scientists can actually see these spin traps at work without having to use expensive electronic devices, such as spectrometers. These spin traps are unique in that they are fat soluble, and thus able to concentrate in the cell plasma membrane, protecting it from free radical damage.

This new class of spin trap is approximately four hundred times stronger than one of the early spin traps, phenylbutyl nitrone (PBN), which I wrote about in my first book, *The Wrinkle Cure*. Chemicals like PBN have been used to treat people who have suffered from stroke. During a stroke, the brain is deprived of oxygen, resulting in a tremendous burst of free radical activity. The cell plasma membrane of the nerve cells becomes damaged, causing an intense inflammatory response. When scientists administered nitrone spin traps to stroke patients, they noticed a significant decrease in the incidence of such problems as loss of speech and paralysis. The azuleneyl nitrone spin traps currently being researched and developed by Dr. Becker have much lower toxicity than previously studied nitrone spin traps. Their greater safety profile combined with their fat solubility have proven to make these new spin traps wonderful anti-inflammatories when applied to the skin.

Azuleneyl nitrones have been shown to have powerful anti-inflammatory powers in a small study looking at their effects when added to a lotion and applied on skin that had been inflamed by ultraviolet light. The new spin traps were applied to the skin three times daily, and the skin redness quickly resolved. The anti-inflammatory action of topically applied spin traps is currently under research for treatment of aging skin. The new spin traps are bound to be an integral part of new antiaging topicals and should be available to the general public by the time you are reading this chapter.

Light Therapy

Dermatologists have used light to treat many dermatologic diseases for years. Exposure to sunlight improves psoriasis and various types of eczema. Certain forms of light therapy, employing ultraviolet light and chemicals called psoralins, have been used to treat certain forms of cancer. Now, light therapy is emerging for the treatment of aging skin.

Laser therapy is, of course, a form of light therapy. The use of lasers to treat aging skin has benefits, however sometimes it has a high price. Lasers cause a certain amount of tissue destruction. Often laser treatments will leave the patient with inflammation, which lasts for weeks or months, that accelerates the aging process. New forms of laser therapy are being developed that cause less tissue destruction, diminishing the inflammatory response.

Other forms of light therapy are proving to be beneficial for the improvement and prevention of aging skin. The visible light from the sun is a mixture of all different colors of the spectrum, and thus appears to be almost white. A rainbow is created when water droplets in the air bend the light, causing the various wavelengths of light to become visible. Blue light, which has been shown to possess some anti-inflammatory capability, is characterized by a wavelength of 400 to 500 nanometers. When blue light is applied to the skin, clinical improvement has been noted. Specifically, when applied to the skin at certain frequencies, lengths of time, and intensities, blue light gives the skin a much smoother appearance. Other frequencies of light in the green range and the red range have also been shown to be beneficial to the skin.

We can expect that visible light therapy, especially of the blue range, will become available to obtain these benefits. Filters can remove all the harmful rays of light and other colors, leaving only the beneficial blue spectrum. Imagine sitting under a special light-filtering beach umbrella in the future. We will be able to enjoy the beach while repairing our skin, which would be a much-welcomed advance. Visible light therapy for the treatment of aging skin is a promising area of research about which you will be hearing more and more.

The Miracle of the Ageless—Electrical and Chemical Stimulation of Muscles for a More Youthful Appearance

One day, a forty-year-old man looks in the mirror and notices that his pectorals and biceps are sagging. Though he would not consider himself vain, he makes a conscious choice to improve his looks by getting into shape. He joins a gym and starts weight training. Day after day, he keeps up the routine, doing curls and bench presses. After six to eight weeks, his strength has increased; he is using heavier weights to get the same resistance. Along with an increase in muscle strength, he notices that his sagging chest and biceps have lifted, toned, and have a pleasingly bulging contour. (As we already know, increased muscle tone shortens the muscles, creating lift and a more youthful appearance. Aging causes a loss of muscle tone that results in the sagging and lengthening of those muscles.)

Would this same forty-year-old man, after looking in the mirror and seeing his sagging chest and arms, have considered calling his plastic surgeon to have those muscles cut, shortened, and sutured to give his chest and arms new tone? I doubt it. Even if he did, those muscles would be stretched taut. They might *appear* firmer, but they would also look unnatural and not so youthful. In addition, he would have done nothing for the underlying problem: weak muscle tissue. As absurd as this scenario is, this is the choice thousands of people are making for their facial muscles every day.

For example, a forty-year-old woman looks in the mirror and notices the deep creases in her forehead and vertical lines between her eyes, caused by the weakening and lengthening of the underlying muscles that results in changes in the overlying skin. Instead of trying to strengthen these muscles, which is guaranteed to result in a more youthful appearance, the woman asks her physician to paralyze the muscles with Botox, one of today's most common cosmetic treatments. Botox has been available for various applications for at least a dozen years and has an excellent safety profile. While paralyzing muscles in the forehead, Botox temporarily relaxes deep creases. It is a quick, easy, and painless procedure. Studies using DMAE technology over a period of six to twelve months have achieved the same effect as Botox in a more natural way, as you have observed in photographs from the Johnson & Johnson DMAE clinical trials.

Although I have always been interested in the positive effects of exercise on muscles, there have been no practical ways to exercise facial muscles. My patients have often asked me about the effectiveness of electrical stimulation to muscles. I had not seen any studies that proved the benefit of electrical-stimulation devices for prevention and reversal of sagging skin. Intrigued by the results of topical DMAE, I thought that perhaps using DMAE with electrical stimulation could produce more dramatic results than DMAE alone.

The electrical-stimulation devices available in today's marketplace are bulky and awkward to use. I wanted to research the effectiveness of electrical muscle stimulation but didn't want to work with one of those unwieldy metal or plastic machines. So I developed an electrical-stimulation glove. Simple and sleek, the glove can easily be slipped on the hand. The tips of the gloves' fingers contain electrodes that can be placed against the skin that lies atop important muscles. An electrical impulse of varying intensity can be applied to these facial muscles simply by using the fingertips, causing repeated contraction of these muscles that, in effect, exercises them.

I designed a study in which the electrical-stimulation glove was used in combination with twice-daily applications of DMAE. The results were dramatic. After three months of using DMAE and electrical stimulation on the face, we observed results that usually took a much longer period of time using DMAE alone. The study proved definitively that electrical stimulation along with the use of topical DMAE greatly reduced sagging in the face, jawline, and neck; reduced wrinkles; and increased skin firmness. Every participant in the study saw a significant return to more youthful contours and a greatly enhanced appearance. The patients who continued to use the device continued to see even more and better benefits.

Full, Youthful Lips

One of the unexpected findings we discovered when using DMAE plus electrical stimulation is an increase in lip fullness, contour, and color. Patients who applied the DMAE lip plumper before doing the electrical stimulation exercises had astounding results. Within three to four months of stimulating the muscles around the mouth, my patients reported, and I observed, gratifying changes. The most surprising finding was that young patients, who had no real signs of facial aging or loss of lip volume, showed an increase in lip size. This means that a person with thin lips could now make them fuller and more beautiful naturally without having to resort to surgery or injection of cosmetic fillers such as collagen. My older patients have reported that, in addition to increased lip volume and contour, strong definition of their lip borders had returned, reducing bleeding and feathering of lipstick.

In addition to having positive effects on underlying musculature, I have observed changes that indicate electrical stimulation is also effective on skin structure itself. Patients with dry skin have noticed that electrical stimulation of the facial muscles has affected sebaceous production, normalizing dry, irritated skin. Long-term use of electrical stimulation causes skin to appear thicker and more youthful, with a vibrant, visible glow. When used in conjunction with DMAE, the electrical stimulation also greatly diminishes dark circles and puffiness.

Clinical observation has confirmed that patients using DMAE plus electrical stimulation can even thicken eyelashes and eyebrows. As we age, hair growth in these areas normally becomes thin and sparse. A male patient using DMAE plus electrical stimulation reported thickened hair growth in the frontal scalp that I cannot confirm upon clinical examination. A larger study will have to be undertaken to explore that exciting possibility.

A number of patients found using the exercise glove for thirty minutes a day too time-consuming and have opted to use topical DMAE alone. I always tell them that using DMAE in conjunction with electrical stimulation produces the best results. The investment of time is minimal when compared to the remarkable changes the technique produces. Patients who have continued to use the electrical stimulation during a period of four to six months have seen optimal results. Electrical stimulation with topical DMAE enhancement will become a realistic and powerful option for maintaining youthful contours, toned appearance, and a radiant complexion with results comparable to cosmetic surgery. I cannot recommend this regimen too highly if you want to turn back the clock and rediscover the face of your youth.

There will always be a place for cosmetic surgery, but we can certainly delay these invasive procedures. Many plastic surgeons are recommending DMAE plus electrical stimulation as a preoperative program, because toned muscles require less surgical correction. If the surgery is less radical, the results not only look more natural but also last longer.

Skin Brightening Agents

Hardly a day goes by without a patient—and it is usually a woman—complaining of darkened spots on the skin, especially on the forehead, cheeks, and chin. This condition, known as melasma, is caused by the interaction of hormones, (for example, estrogen in the skin, which is why this condition often occurs in pregnant and oral contraceptive–using women) and sunlight. The current available treatments of melasma are less than satisfactory, and consist of applying topical bleaching agents like hydroquinone, Retin-A, and kogic acid. These therapies require a fairly lengthy period of treatment and are not totally effective.

As discussed in Chapter Five, Asian skin may be characterized by a lack of radiance. Many of my Asian patients are constantly searching for skin-brightening agents. Many of my darker-skinned patients, Latino and African-American, also suffer from dark patches if there is the slightest bit of inflammation present in their skin. Topical alpha lipoic acid has been of some help, but I have not been completely satisfied with the results.

A fortuitous accident—well before I entered medical school—gave me the clue to an excellent skin-brightening treatment. I have always taken large doses of vitamin C and had discovered pure, powdered L-ascorbic acid that I mixed in water and drank several times a day. Because vitamin C is extremely unstable, this solution must be mixed fresh each time it is taken. My habit was to mix my vitamin C in the kitchen and carry the glass to my bedroom upstairs.

After a while, I was dismayed to notice some bright orange and yellow spots on my new carpet. I tried to remove the spots with carpet cleaner to no avail. I called the carpet manufacturer who sent someone over to inspect and clean the carpet. He told me that the carpet was not defective and that I was somehow exposing the carpet to a bleaching agent that was taking the color out of the fiber. I was baffled. It was time to start some detective work. I soon noticed that the spots formed a trail from the kitchen, upstairs, and to the bedroom. I occasionally spilled vitamin C solution as I carried my glass upstairs. The vitamin C was bleaching a carpet that was guaranteed to be colorfast! I had never known that vitamin C was such a powerful bleaching agent. But how could I harness this power to help my patients? (As you will remember, the problem with vitamin C is that it is not practical for use on the skin since it is extremely unstable and very irritating.) I needed to find a substance that possessed vitamin C's outstanding bleaching abilities *without* the irritating side effects.

Alpha hydroxy tetronic Acid

The alpha hydroxy tetronic acid molecule is very similar to that of vitamin C except that it is missing a side chain of atoms. Because of this configuration, the antioxidant power of tetronic acid is even more powerful than vitamin C!

I believed that tetronic acid could be an effective brightening agent for the skin. Tetronic acid is nontoxic and is much less irritating than the L-ascorbic acid form of vitamin C. I incorporated alpha hydroxy tetronic acid into a topical lotion and applied it to a small spot on the back of my hand. Much to my delight, in a couple of hours, the skin in the area where the cream had been applied was brighter than the skin on the rest of my hand. Alpha hydroxy tetronic acid appeared to be an ideal skin-brightening agent. A larger study performed by a plastic surgery group showed that alpha hydroxy tetronic acid confirmed my observation. Alpha hydroxy tetronic acid is faster acting than any brightener that has been discovered to date.

When spread evenly over large areas of the skin, tetronic acid gives the skin a brighter appearance. This has become extremely popular among my Asian patients, since alpha hydroxy tetronic acid effectively eliminates the sallowness that can occur in this skin type. It is effective for *all* shades of skin. Alpha hydroxy tetronic acid can be mixed with more traditional brightening agents for synergistic effects. I am convinced that tetronic acid alone—without the additions—is an ideal agent for brightening skin and effectively eliminating troublesome dark and/or light areas. I feel confident in predicting that alpha hydroxy tetronic acid will be the new skin-brightening agent of the future.

Telomerase—A Shot at Immortality

A cell has a finite life span. When a cell becomes old, it stops dividing, a process known as senescence. The single exception to this rule is cancer cells. They are immortal. The irony is that the only immortal cell is one that brings an end to our lives. Researchers have focused on the fact that normal cells cannot divide indefinitely. They have associated the inability of the cell to divide to a shortening of a portion of the chromosome called the telomere. Each time a cell divides, a small portion at the end of the chromosome breaks off. This shortening continues until there is nothing left to divide. Scientists have even used the length of the telomere at the end of the chromosome to determine someone's chronological age, sort of the reverse of counting tree rings.

The reason cancer cells divide forever and do not become senescent is that they contain an enzyme called telomerase. This enzyme can add DNA to the end of the telomere, lengthening it and allowing the cell to divide indefinitely without ever reaching senescence. Researchers have been looking for a way to introduce the enzyme telomerase into healthy cells to increase their life spans. Jerry Shay, Ph.D., of the University of Texas Southwestern Medical Center, introduced the enzyme telomerase into the cells in our body that make collagen. He found that these cells, known as fibroblasts, continued to divide without reaching senescence. Since Dr. Shay's studies, more research has shown that cells can divide indefinitely without becoming cancerous. And researchers are studying ways to remove telomerase from cancer cells to make cancer mortal, so that the cells age and die.

We know how to introduce telomerase into skin cells by using a topical lotion containing liposomes. The liposomes fuse to the cell membrane, allowing telomerase to enter the cell. Telomerase creams are currently being developed, and will be available in five to ten years, providing us with a super antiaging cream. I intend to watch this area of research with great interest in the hope that we may have a practical product in the near future.

Hormone Replacement Therapy

Hormone Replacement Therapy (HRT) is an area that is currently being explored by clinicians and research physicians as an age-management strategy. Supplementation with any of the youth hormones such as testosterone, estrogen, DHEA, or Human Growth Hormone (HGH) results in decreased levels of cortisol, the death hormone. Women have received HRT for a number of years and now we are seeing men supplementing testosterone as they age.

Another type of hormone strategy for both men and women, which is highly controversial, is supplemental human growth hormone. In the first study, injectable human growth hormone was given to men over a six-month period. They showed a remarkable increase in cognitive function including memory, increase in muscle mass, decrease in body fat, a healthier heart, lungs and kidneys, increased bone density, elevation of mood and energy and an increased libido. As exciting as these results were, there was a downside. Subsequent studies using injectable growth hormone at similar doses to the first study found unacceptable side effects.

These studies were extended to a period of a year or longer and researchers realized that prolonged supplementation could induce diabetes, arthritis, or carpal tunnel syndrome, making these results very disappointing.

Some of the more recent studies have used much lower doses of injectable growth hormone at a greater frequency to better mimic the way human growth hormone is secreted by our pituitary gland. These studies reveal a much lower side effect profile, achieving some of the benefits seen at higher doses.

Supplementation with injectable human growth hormone is still very experimental and we have not accumulated enough data to assure its safety. When physicians administer HGH to their patients, they monitor the therapeutic levels by a metabolite of the hormone called Insulin Growth Factor 1 (IGF-1). Human growth hormone cannot be measured directly because it is detectable in the blood for only a few minutes. However, IGF-1 is a pro-inflammatory molecule that is seen in high levels in older, more sedentary people and in cancer patients, and there is a strong correlation between IGF-1 levels and cancer risk. Thus, recent developments in transdermal delivery of HGH provide the therapeutic benefits without the risk of IGF-1.

Another very new and exciting strategy for growth hormone supplementation is to use amino acids or small peptides to trigger the body's own release of human growth hormone from our pituitary. This is a much safer method because we have normal feedback mechanisms and controls over a hormone when it is being produced by our own bodies. In addition, when these growth hormone-releasing peptides are administered along with other peptides that have inflammatory activity, such as sex hormone-releasing peptide, we see an increase in growth hormone levels with a seemingly contradictory decrease in levels of IGF-1. Some of these newer products can be applied to the skin in a lotion form, which is then absorbed resulting in an increase in circulating growth hormone. One of the criticisms for this method is that the product initially works but then the pituitary becomes depleted of its growth hormone stores and subsequent use is not effective. This controversy will have to be settled by the clinicians and physicians currently administering this treatment.

I have done extensive research on transdermal delivery systems for many types of medications and nutrients. This has led to a clinical study wherein insulin can be delivered to diabetics by simply rubbing an insulin containing cream utilizing my transdermal technology rather than use of hypodermic syringes and needles. Delivering nutrients such as amino acids and vitamins using the transdermal system is exciting and almost limitless. For example, I have treated patients with simple amino acids to relieve stress, increase libido, or raise critical levels of glutathione in several cases.

Thymic Hormones

The thymus is responsible for the function of a large portion of our immune system. Located in the chest, this gland is most active throughout our teen years and begins to shrink as we enter adulthood. The thymus produces a series of hormones that have been the subject of thorough investigation since the 1960s. In addition to affecting the competency of the immune system, these hormones are active in all areas of our bodies. They have even been shown to work in the brain to affect mood. Extracts of the thymus gland—called thymosins—have been studied. We all remember the story of the boy in the bubble who had to remain isolated from the world because he did not have a competent immune system. In the 1970s, children with other types of life-threatening immune deficiencies were treated with a thymic preparation. This preparation, thymosin fraction 5, is important in the regulation and function of immune cells called lymphocytes. Allan Goldstein, Ph.D., formerly of the University of Texas and now professor and chairman of the Department of Biochemistry and Molecular Biology at the George Washington University School of Medicine, was responsible for much of the work done with fraction 5. Fraction 5, which consists of twenty-three different peptides, was first administered to children with severely compromised immune systems to restore T-cell functions. Fraction 5 has also been shown to act in a way similar to growth hormone. This is an exciting field of study for antiaging, because it means that fraction 5 can affect cellular growth and activity. And fraction 5 shows virtually no toxicity.

Dr. Goldstein continued his research and found that one of the biologically active peptides, which was part of fraction 5, showed even greater promise. This peptide, designated thymosin beta 4, shows tremendous potential in the field of antiaging. We have all become familiar with the importance of inflammation in the aging process and those diseases related to aging. My research has centered upon a quest for powerful anti-inflammatories, and thymosin beta 4 looks extremely promising. We all know that cortisone, a medication used routinely by doctors, has powerful anti-inflammatory effects. However, the resulting negative side effects limit its use to very short periods of time. Research shows that thymosin beta 4 is produced by cells in the body when cortisone is administered. Thymosin beta 4 is a powerful anti-inflammatory, and we may be able to use it in place of the very powerful but dangerous steroids, thus avoiding side effects.

One of the most sensitive areas of the body is the eye, and the thin lens covering the eye (the cornea) is vulnerable to damage. Thymosin beta 4 has been used in animal trials to heal the cornea after injury. It was shown that this therapy rapidly decreased inflammation and promoted corneal healing in a matter of a few days. Thymosin beta 4 has also been tested on wounds and it has been shown to rapidly accelerate wound closure. It even has worked on chronic wounds in diabetic animals who have difficulty healing as a result of compromised blood circulation. Although clinical studies have not yet begun, the use of thymosin beta 4 for treatment of aging skin should show great success. Because we know that inflammation, whether from sunlight or metabolism, damages the skin very much like any other wound, the use of this powerful anti-inflammatory molecule may result in a tremendous breakthrough.

The foregoing has been just a brief review of the exciting developments in antiaging skin care you can look forward to in the very near future. In the meantime, you are now armed with the knowledge of the most up-to-the-minute treatments and techniques available to restore freshness and suppleness to your skin and to retard the development of lines, wrinkles, and sagging. When you follow my 28-Day Wrinkle-Free Program, you will discover the key to new levels of energy and radiance.

By taking care of your body's needs for proper nourishment, activity, and calm, you will live longer and the quality of your life will be better. If you consume the right food and supplements and care for your skin with products that reflect the latest in scientific know-how to fight inflammation, your skin will look as great as you feel. Nothing contributes to your appearance more than a glowing, supple, smooth complexion.

I hope that you find the program as rewarding as have so many of my patients. It gives me great pleasure to set you on the right path to being wrinkle free for life. I am sure you will be equally delighted when you experience the extraordinary transformation my program will accomplish for you.

Appendix A
RECIPES FOR THE PERRICONE PROGRAM

The Perricone Wrinkle-Free Program is easy to follow and requires very little in the way of cooking or special preparation. To fight free radicals, reverse signs of aging, and stay on a healthy path for life, it helps to learn a few simple recipes to add variety and zest to the regimen.

My 28-Day Program calls for protein and vegetables every day. If you prefer to keep cooking to a minimum, you may simply broil the fish or chicken and steam the vegetables. If you want to shake it up a bit, use one of the following recipes. For example, the Day 4 dinner calls for brussels sprouts. You can either steam a few heads on the stove or in the microwave or you can follow the simple recipe for Oven-Roasted Brussels Sprouts with Apples.

Vegetables—Nature's Antioxidant Storehouse

Grilled Asparagus

½ pound fresh asparagus
1 teaspoon extra virgin olive oil
Freshly ground black pepper
1 teaspoon finely chopped fresh parsley

1. Place asparagus on a plate, drizzle with olive oil, and season with pepper to taste.

2. Roll asparagus to coat each stalk with oil.

3. Place on very hot ridged grill or in a broiler, and cook until stalks start to brown. Turn and cook other side.

4. Remove to serving plate and garnish with parsley.

YIELD: 2 SERVINGS.

Note: Cold leftover asparagus is great in a salad.

Sautéed Zucchini or Summer Squash

2 cloves garlic, slivered
2 teaspoons extra virgin olive oil
2 medium zucchini, sliced lengthwise
1 tablespoon fresh dill

1. In 8-inch pan quickly sauté the garlic in the olive oil over medium heat.

2. Add the sliced zucchini and toss until covered with oil and garlic.

3. Add fresh dill, lower the heat, and cover pan for a few minutes to cook through.

YIELD: 3 SERVINGS.

Oven-Roasted Brussels Sprouts with Apples

1 pint brussels sprouts, cleaned and left whole
1 apple, peeled, cored, and cut into eighths
1 teaspoon extra virgin olive oil

1. Preheat oven to 375° F.

2. In a large bowl, toss brussels sprouts, apple, and oil together.

3. Cover a cookie sheet with aluminum foil; spread apple–brussels sprouts mixture evenly.

4. Roast uncovered for 20 minutes.

YIELD: 2 SERVINGS.

Oven-Roasted Cauliflower

> 1 head cauliflower, separated into florets
> 1 teaspoon extra virgin olive oil
> 1 tablespoon finely chopped fresh parsley

1. Preheat oven to 375° F.

2. In a bowl toss cauliflower and olive oil.

3. Cover a cookie sheet with aluminum foil; spread cauliflower evenly over it.

4. Roast for 15 minutes. Turn cauliflower pieces and continue cooking for another 15 minutes.

> YIELD: 4 SERVINGS.

Roasted Eggplant

> 3 skinny purple eggplants
> 2 teaspoon extra virgin olives oil
> Freshly ground black pepper
> 3 cloves garlic
> 2 fresh plum tomatoes, chopped, or one 8-ounce can of
>   chopped plum tomatoes
> 1 tablespoon grated Parmesan cheese
> 1 tablespoon dried oregano

1. Preheat oven to 375° F.

2. Cut off stem end of each eggplant; slice into 2-inch chunks and place in a casserole dish.

3. Sprinkle with olive oil and top with freshly ground black pepper.

4. Cut each garlic clove in half and nestle among the eggplant pieces.

5. Layer tomatoes atop eggplant and garlic.

6. Top with cheese.

7. Roast for 15 minutes. Turn and continue cooking for another 15 minutes.

8. Top with oregano.

> YIELD: 2 SERVINGS.

Sautéed Spinach

> 2 pounds fresh spinach
> 1 tablespoon extra virgin olive oil
> 1 clove garlic, minced or extruded through a garlic press
> Juice of ½ fresh lemon
> Red pepper flakes (optional)

1. Thoroughly wash spinach leaves; remove stems.

2. Heat oil in sauté pan.

3. Add garlic and cook briefly.

4. Toss spinach in hot oil-garlic mixture, cover, and cook until wilted (should take only a minute or two).

5. Remove from heat, place in serving bowl, and sprinkle with freshly squeezed lemon juice.

6. Sprinkle with red pepper flakes (if desired).

> YIELD: 4 SERVINGS.

Note: Also works with escarole, broccoli rabe, and other greens.

Salads—The Power of Raw Foods

A plate of raw vegetables lightly dressed with lemon juice, garlic, and a bit of olive oil offers great antioxidant protection. The recipes that follow are just a sample of what can be done with the bounty of fresh, colorful vegetables available in the produce aisle.

Mediterranean Tomato Salad

> 2 large tomatoes, thinly sliced
> 1 tablespoon fresh chopped basil
> 1 small red onion, thinly sliced
> 1 clove garlic, finely chopped
> 1 tablespoon extra virgin olive oil

Juice of one large lemon
Freshly ground black pepper

1. Place tomato slices on serving plate.

2. Arrange basil and onion atop tomato slices.

3. In a bowl mix garlic, olive oil, and lemon juice and pour over vegetables.

4. Sprinkle with ground pepper to taste. For fullest flavor, prepare ahead of time and let mixture marinate for about an hour before serving—although this still tastes great when served immediately.

YIELD: 4 SERVINGS.

Mediterranean Chopped Salad

1 cucumber, peeled and diced into ¼-inch cubes
1 red bell pepper, diced into ¼-inch cubes
3 stalks celery, diced into ¼-inch cubes
1 cup cherry tomatoes, quartered
2 tablespoons chopped red onion
2 tablespoons finely chopped fresh parsley
1 tablespoon freshly squeezed lemon juice
6 black olives, pitted and quartered
2 ounces crumbled feta cheese
2 tablespoons extra virgin olive oil

Mix all ingredients together in large nonmetallic bowl and serve.

YIELD: 4 SERVINGS.

Pacific Rim Salad

3 cups napa cabbage, thinly sliced
1 cup snow peas, slivered
1 red bell pepper, slivered
¼ cup scallions, chopped

2 tablespoons chopped fresh cilantro

2 tablespoons lime juice

2 tablespoons chopped green onions

½ tablespoon low-sodium soy sauce

¾ teaspoon grated fresh ginger

1 clove crushed garlic

1 teaspoon sesame oil

2 tablespoons extra virgin olive oil

1 tablespoon hazelnuts, chopped

1. Toss together all cabbage, snow peas, bell pepper, scallions, and cilantro.

2. Whisk together lime juice, onions, soy sauce, ginger, garlic, and sesame and olive oils.

3. Pour over salad and toss.

4. Top with hazelnuts.

YIELD: 4 SERVINGS.

Italian Summer Salad

½ cup cherry tomatoes

1 green bell pepper, slivered

1 head romaine lettuce, torn into bite-size pieces

½ cup finely chopped fennel

¼ cup red onion, sliced into rings

6 black olives, pitted and sliced

4 radishes, thinly sliced

2 tablespoons extra virgin olive oil

Juice of one lemon

1 clove garlic, crushed

1 pinch dried oregano

Freshly ground black pepper

1. Mix together first seven ingredients.

2. Whisk together olive oil, lemon juice, garlic, and oregano.

3. Pour dressing over salad, toss lightly, season with freshly ground black pepper to taste.

YIELD: 4 SERVINGS.

Chickpea Salad

15-ounce-can chickpeas, drained and rinsed
1 clove garlic, crushed
1 tablespoon extra virgin olive oil
1 teaspoon fresh rosemary, chopped

1. Mix all ingredients together in nonmetallic bowl.

2. Let mixture sit for at least one hour at room temperature to allow flavors to mingle.

YIELD: 4 SERVINGS.

Cuban Black Bean Salad

15-ounce can black beans, drained and rinsed
½ cup yellow bell pepper, chopped
½ cup red bell pepper, chopped
½ cup chopped celery
2 tablespoons red onion, chopped
1 tablespoon chopped fresh parsley
2 tablespoons freshly squeezed lemon juice
1 clove garlic, crushed
¼ teaspoon ground cumin
2 tablespoons extra virgin olive oil

1. Toss together beans, yellow and red bell peppers, celery, onion, and parsley.

2. Whisk together lemon juice, garlic, and cumin.

3. Lightly toss salad with dressing and serve.

YIELD: 4 SERVINGS.

Three-Bean Salad

15-ounce can chickpeas
15-ounce can kidney beans
15-ounce can black beans
2 cloves garlic, minced
Juice of one freshly squeezed lemon
2 tablespoons extra virgin olive oil

1. Mix beans together in a salad bowl.
2. In a cup combine garlic, lemon juice, and olive oil.
3. Toss beans with dressing and serve.
   YIELD: 8 SERVINGS.
Note: For easy and delicious variations, add bell peppers, onion, celery, parsley, or other seasoning.

Soup—A Delicious Bowl of Antioxidants

Mediterranean Chicken-Vegetable Soup

2 cups chopped onions
3 cloves garlic, chopped
2 tablespoons chopped fresh parsley
1 tablespoon extra virgin olive oil
2 cups shredded savoy cabbage
1 cup green beans, cut into ¼ inch pieces
½ cup diced celery
1 cup canned navy beans, drained and rinsed
1 cup canned diced tomatoes
1 cup diced zucchini
2 boneless skinless chicken breasts
6 cups chicken broth, add more as desired
1 cup shredded fresh spinach
Pesto (see page 234 for recipe)

1. Sauté onions, garlic, parsley, and olive oil over medium heat.

2. Add cabbage and cook until softened.

3. Transfer to soup pot. Add green beans, celery, navy beans, tomatoes, zucchini, broth, and chicken.

4. Simmer for 30 minutes over low heat. Keep lid on to preserve flavor and to avoid losing nutrients in the steam.

5. Add spinach and cook on low heat for another minute.

6. Ladle into bowls and top each serving with 1 tablespoon of pesto.

YIELD: 8 SERVINGS.

Cuban Black Bean Soup

¼ cup extra virgin olive oil

½ cup chopped onion

½ medium green bell pepper, chopped

1 teaspoon dried parsley (or 1 tablespoon fresh)

4 cloves garlic, minced

1½ quarts low-salt chicken broth

5 ounces dry black beans, sorted, rinsed, and soaked
  overnight

½ teaspoon dried oregano leaves

½ teaspoon ground cumin

½ teaspoon cayenne pepper

1. In a large, heavy soup pot, heat oil over medium-high heat. Add onion, green pepper, parsley, and garlic and sauté for 6 minutes.

2. Add chicken broth, black beans, oregano, cumin, and cayenne pepper.

3. Bring to a boil. Reduce heat to low and let soup simmer for 55 minutes or until beans are tender. Remove from heat and let soup cool.

4. Purée about half the soup, 2 cups at a time, in a blender at low speed or in a food processor.

5. Return purée to pot, stirring into remaining soup. Stir over low heat until heated.

YIELD: 4–6 SERVINGS.

Chicken-Vegetable Soup

3 pounds skinless, boneless chicken breasts
1 red or green bell pepper
1 onion, diced
1 cup raw or frozen broccoli
1 cup raw mushrooms
2 stalks celery, diced
4 sprigs fresh parsley
2 bay leaves
½ teaspoon thyme
2 tablespoons chopped fresh dill
2 whole cloves garlic
1 tablespoon extra virgin olive oil
15-ounce can pinto beans

1. Cut up chicken and place in large soup pot; add enough water to cover.

2. Bring to a boil, then simmer uncovered 35 minutes.

3. While chicken is simmering, lightly sauté pepper, onions, broccoli, mushrooms, celery, herbs, and garlic in oil.

4. Add sautéed vegetable mixture to soup, and cook 1½ hours covered.

5. Add beans for final 15 minutes of cooking.

YIELD: 8 SERVINGS.

Manhattan Clam Chowder

2 cups finely chopped onions
1 cup chopped celery
2 tablespoons extra virgin olive oil
4 cups clam broth
1 teaspoon thyme
1 bay leaf

35-ounce can peeled, chopped tomatoes
½ cup chopped fresh parsley
2 15-ounce cans chopped clams

1. Sauté onions and celery in olive oil over low heat until tender.

2. Add everything except the clams and simmer partially covered for 30 minutes.

3. Add clams and cook additional 5 minutes over low heat.

YIELD: 4 SERVINGS.

Fish—The Ultimate Antiaging Protein Source

I look forward to a beautiful piece of broiled salmon in the morning. My three-year-old daughter loves it, too, and often climbs into my lap to gobble up my breakfast.

Fish is wonderful simply broiled with a squeeze of lemon juice, but it also responds well to a variety of cooking methods and seasonings. On the Wrinkle-Free Program, you can savor all sorts of fish prepared in a number of tempting ways—from salmon teriyaki to steamed mussels to sole baked in foil.

Salmon with Pesto

4- to 6-ounce salmon filet
2 tablespoons pesto (see page 234 for recipe)
3 cherry tomatoes, halved

1. Preheat oven to 375° F.

2. Cover a cookie sheet with aluminum foil.

3. Place salmon on foil and spread with a thin layer of pesto.

4. Top with tomato halves.

5. Bake 20 minutes.

YIELD: 1 SERVING.

Salmon Teriyaki

2 tablespoons low-sodium soy sauce
1 tablespoon chopped fresh ginger
½ cup minced scallions
1 teaspoon minced garlic
8 ounce salmon filet

1. Whisk together soy sauce, ginger, scallions, and garlic in a nonmetallic bowl.
2. Place salmon filet in shallow dish and cover with soy-ginger sauce. Allow to marinate for 30 minutes.
3. Cover baking sheet with foil.
4. Place fish on foil and top with any remaining marinade.
5. Broil 5 to 7 minutes.
YIELD: 1 LARGE OR 2 SMALL SERVINGS.

Garlic Shrimp

8 cloves garlic, slivered
1 tablespoon extra virgin olive oil
⅓ cup freshly squeezed lemon juice
1 pinch cayenne pepper
1 pound large shrimp
¼ cup chopped parsley

1. Combine garlic with lemon juice, cayenne pepper, and shrimp.
2. Marinate shrimp for 1 hour in refrigerator.
3. Heat olive oil and sauté shrimp 3 minutes each side.
4. Sprinkle with parsley and serve.
YIELD: 3–4 SERVINGS.

Sole Baked in Foil

Three 6-ounce fillets of sole
Large tomato, thinly sliced
12 fresh basil leaves
1 tablespoon extra virgin olive oil

1. Preheat oven to 425° F.
2. Place fish on 12-inch-square piece of aluminum foil.
3. Top with tomato and basil.
4. Drizzle with olive oil.
5. Fold foil over fish to form an envelope; crimp edges to close.
6. Bake on cookie sheet for 15 minutes.
   YIELD: 3 SERVINGS.

Scallops with Garlic and Parsley

1 tablespoon extra virgin olive oil
2 cloves garlic, finely chopped
1 pound scallops, drained
2 tablespoons chopped fresh parsley

1. Sauté oil and garlic in oil; add scallops.
2. Sauté scallops until lightly browned; turn onto serving plate.
3. Sprinkle with parsley.
   YIELD: 3–4 SERVINGS.

Steamed Mussels

3 pounds fresh mussels
1 tablespoon extra virgin olive oil
3 tablespoons finely chopped shallots
4 cloves garlic, sliced
1 cup dry white wine
4 tablespoons chopped fresh parsley

1. Scrub and rinse mussels in clean, cold water.
2. Heat oil in two-quart saucepan.
3. Add shallots, garlic and sauté until translucent.
4. Gently add mussels.
5. Pour on white wine and parsley.
6. Cover pan and cook 5 minutes until mussels open. Discard any mussels that do not open.

YIELD: 4 SERVINGS.

Poultry—Another Great Protein Source

Grilled Chicken Breasts

1 teaspoon extra virgin olive oil
1 teaspoon freshly squeezed lemon juice
1 clove garlic, slivered
1 tablespoon chopped fresh parsley
1 boneless, skinless whole chicken breast, split in two and flattened

1. Whisk together olive oil, lemon juice, garlic, and parsley.
2. Pour over chicken breasts and marinate in refrigerator for two hours.
3. Cook on grill pan or broiler for 5 minutes each side.

YIELD: 2 SERVINGS.

Chicken Teriyaki

1 tablespoon low-sodium soy sauce
1 teaspoon Chinese sesame oil
1 teaspoon grated fresh ginger
1 clove garlic, chopped
1 boneless, skinless whole chicken breast, split and flattened

1. Whisk together all the ingredients except the chicken.

2. Pour over chicken, cover with plastic wrap, and marinate in refrigerator for at least four hours.

3. Preheat broiler for 5 minutes.

4. Place chicken on aluminum-foil-covered cookie sheet.

5. Broil 4 inches from flame for 3 minutes each side, or until done.

YIELD: 2 SERVINGS.

Middle Eastern Chicken Kebobs

1 tablespoon extra virgin olive oil

½ teaspoon ground cumin

½ teaspoon ground coriander

½ teaspoon ground turmeric

1 tablespoon finely chopped fresh parsley

2 tablespoons freshly squeezed lemon juice

1 large clove garlic, minced

1 boneless, skinless whole chicken breast, cut into 1-inch chunks

4 green onions, cleaned and cut into 2-inch pieces

1. Combine olive oil, spices, lemon juice, and garlic.

2. Pour over chicken cubes, stir, cover with plastic wrap, and marinate in the refrigerator for at least 1 hour.

3. Thread chicken on skewers, alternating with pieces of green onion.

4. Grill for 4 minutes on each side under hot broiler.

YIELD: 3 SERVINGS.

Perfect Roast Turkey Breast

3 pound boneless turkey breast

2 tablespoons extra virgin olive oil

3 teaspoons dried thyme

Freshly ground black pepper

1 pound onions cut into quarters

½ cup low-sodium chicken broth

1. Preheat oven to 375° F.

2. Rub turkey breast with one tablespoon of olive oil and massage with thyme and pepper.

3. Toss onions with remaining oil and place in roasting pan.

4. Put turkey breast on top of onions; add chicken broth.

5. Roast in oven for one hour or until meat thermometer registers 170° F. Baste occasionally with pan juices.

YIELD: 7–8 SERVINGS.

The following is a delicious accompaniment to grilled poultry or fish.

Basil Pesto

¼ cup pine nuts

3 large cloves garlic

1½ cups fresh basil leaves

2 tablespoons grated fresh Parmesan cheese

1 tablespoon grated Romano cheese

½ cup extra virgin olive oil

Put pine nuts and garlic in food processor and process until minced. Add basil and cheese; process until finely minced. With processor on, slowly pour oil through food chute; process until well blended. Spoon into small container and store in refrigerator.

YIELD: ½ CUP.

Appendix B
RESOURCES

Acne Products containing anti-inflammatory antiaging ingredients
Clinical Creations, LLC (888-823-7837; www.clinicalcreations.com)
Nu Skin

Topical antiaging anti-inflammatory products

VITAMIN C ESTER PRODUCTS
Clinical Creations, LLC (888-823-7837; www.clinicalcreations.com)
Nordstrom, Nordstrom Beauty Hotline (800-7BEAUTY)
Sephora stores (1-877-SEPHORA)
Selected Saks Fifth Avenue stores
Jan Marini Skin Research, Inc.: through doctors' offices only

ALPHA LIPOIC ACID PRODUCTS
Clinical Creations, LLC (888-823-7837; www.clinicalcreations.com)
Nordstrom, Nordstrom Beauty Hotline (800-7BEAUTY)
Sephora stores (1-877-SEPHORA)
Selected Saks Fifth Avenue stores
Selected plastic surgeons' and dermatologists' offices
CamoCare products

PRODUCTS CONTAINING DMAE (NTP COMPLEX)
Clinical Creations, LLC (888-823-7837, www.clinicalcreations.com)
Nordstrom, Nordstrom Beauty Hotline (800-7BEAUTY)

Sephora stores (1-877-SEPHORA)
Selected Saks Fifth Avenue Stores
RoC
Jan Marini Skin Research Inc., through physicians only

PRODUCTS CONTAINING OLIVE OIL POLYPHENOLS
Clinical Creations, LLC (888-823-7837; www.clinicalcreations. com)
Nu Skin

PRODUCTS CONTAINING PHOSPHATIDYL CHOLINE
Clinical Creations, LLC (888-823-7837; www.clinicalcreations. com)
Nu Skin

PRODUCTS CONTAINING TOCOTRIENOLS
Clinical Creations, LLC (888-823-7837; www.clinicalcreations. com)

PRODUCTS FOR DIMINISHING THE APPEARANCE OF SCARS
Clinical Creations, LLC (888-823-7837; www.clinicalcreations. com)

ALPHA HYDROXY ACID PRODUCTS
Aqua Glycolic brand (Merz Pharmaceuticals); available in pharmacies
Pond's Age Defying Complex; available in pharmacies
Avon Anew All-in-One Intensive Complex
Jan Marini Skin Research Inc., through physicians only
Glyderm: (800-321-4576), M. D. Forte (800-253-9499); Murad (physicians/aestheticians) (800-33MURAD)

COENZYME Q10 CREAM
Beiersdorf
Nivea Visage Wrinkle Control Q10
Juvena

Cleansers

Cetaphil, liquid and bar (Galderma)
Dove Beauty Bar (Unilever)
Oil of Olay Beauty Bar (Procter & Gamble)
Basis Sensitive Skin Bar
Neutrogena Non-Drying Cleansing Lotion
N.V. Perricone M.D. Nutritive Cleanser
N.V. Perricone M.D. Olive Oil Polyphenol Cleanser

Moisturizers

OILY SKIN
Alpha-Hydrox Oil-Free Formula (Neoteric Cosmetics, Inc.)
Prescriptives All You Need for Oily Skin (Estée Lauder)

NORMAL TO DRY SKIN
Neutrogena Healthy Skin Face Lotion
Oil of Olay Daily UV Protectant Beauty Fluid (Procter & Gamble)
Pen-Kera Lotion (B. F. Ascher)
Eucerin Face Cream (Beiersdorf)

Sunscreens

Minimum recommendation is SPF-15. An abbreviated list of companies
offering excellent sunscreens:

Westwood-Squibb—PreSun products
Hawaiian Tropic—Suncare products
Sun Pharmaceuticals—Banana Boat products
Schering-Plough—Coppertone products
Procter & Gamble—Oil of Olay UV Protective lotions
Estée Lauder—In the Sun products
Fisher Pharmaceuticals—Ultrasol
Beiersdorf—Eucerin Daily Facial Lotion
Avon—Sunseekers

Copper Peptide Complex Skin Cream

Skin Biology, Inc. (800-405-1912)
Protect & Restore Skin Renewal Cream

Vitamin and Nutritionals Supplements

Multivitamin packets containing entire Perricone Program:

Clinical Creations Skin and Total Body Nutritional Supplements (888-823-7837 or www.clinicalcreations.com)

Optimum Health: Outstanding supplement line (800-228-1507)

Bronson Pharmaceuticals: A complete line of high-quality vitamins and minerals at excellent prices (800-235-3200 or fax 801-756-5739)

Life Extension Foundation (1-800-544-4440). This is a great source of high-quality, hard-to-find supplements.

Body Fat Metabolizer Supplement Packets

Clinical Creations, LLC (888-823-7837; www.clinicalcreations.com)

Sephora

Nordstrom's

Selected natural food stores

Wild Alaskan Salmon

Vital Choice Seafood: (800-608-4825) delivers premium wild Alaskan sockeye ("red") salmon products via Federal Express or UPS at affordable prices.

Alaskan Seafood Marketing Institute

Information on Hormone Supplementation

The Wisdom of Menopause: Creating Physical and Emotional Health and Healing During the Change, by Christiane Northrup, M.D. (New York: Bantam Books, 2001).

Antiaging Doctors

American Academy of Anti-Aging Medicine (773-528-4333)

Directory of Innovative Doctors, published by the Life Extension Foundation (800-544-4440)

Topical Glutathione

Clinical Creations, LLC (888-823-7837; www.clinicalcreations.com)

Low Glycemic Nutritional Protein Bars (containing key antiaging nutrients (DMAE, Alpha Lipoic Acid, Vitamin C Ester, etc.)

Clinical Creations, LLC (888-823-7837; www.clinicalcreations. com)

Electrical Muscle Stimulator Glove for Face

Clinical Creations, LLC (888-823-7837; www.clinicalcreations. com)

Electronic Muscle Stimulator for Body

Flextone, Ltd., PMB 313 2457A South Hiawassee Road, Orlando, FL 32835 (Order line: 1-877-355-7416; customer service: 1-888-231-2216)

Meditative/Inspirational Books to Help Lower Stress Levels

A New You, by Catherine Galasso. Avon, Mass.: Adams Media.

The Healing Power of Pets: Harnessing the Ability of Pets to Make and Keep People Happy and Healthy by Marty Becker, D.V.M. New York: Hyperion, 2002.

The Four Agreements: A Practical Guide to Personal Freedom by don Miguel Ruiz. San Rafael, Calif.: Amber-Allen Publishing, 1997.

Topical Human Growth Hormone Treatment

Consult your physician

For more information www.balancederm.com

Transdermal Delivery Systems

Transdermal Delivery Systems for Stress Relief

Transdermal Delivery Systems for Increased Libido

Transdermal Delivery Systems for Increased Energy

Clinical Creations, LLC (888-823-7837; www.clinicalcreations. com)

Appendix C
GLOSSARY

ACETYLCHOLINE: a neurotransmitter that causes muscles to contract.

ALDEHYDE: inflammatory chemical produced during the metabolism of alcoholic beverages.

ALPHA HYDROXY ACID: natural exfoliating acid that has anti-inflammatory properties derived from fruit, milk, and sugarcane.

ALPHA LIPOIC ACID: a powerful antioxidant that is both water and fat soluble.

ANTIOXIDANTS: substances that prevent or reverse the development of free radicals.

AP-1: a transcription factor activated by sunlight that promotes the secretion of a collagen-digesting enzyme called metalloproteinase.

ARACHIDONIC ACID: inflammatory compound, produced by the cells in response to the presence of free radicals, that sets into play a cascade of inflammatory events.

ASCORBYL PALMITATE: fat-soluble form of vitamin C. Also known as vitamin C ester.

BASAL LAYER: the bottom layer of the epidermis that produces new skin cells.

CATECHINS: compounds that stabilize collagen and prevent capillary fragility.

CELL PLASMA MEMBRANE: outer layer of a cell where free radicals do the most damage.

COLLAGEN: the protein fibers that give the skin strength and flexibility.

COLLAGENASE: enzyme produced by the cells in response to free radicals. It damages collagen fibers, creating microscarring that leads to wrinkles.

CYTOKINE: inflammatory peptide produced by lymphocytes in response to free radicals and other agents.

CYTOSOL: the watery interior of the cell.

DERMIS: the lower layer of the skin that contains nerve endings, sweat glands, as well as collagen and elastin fibers.

DMAE (DIMETHYLAMINOETHANOL): antioxidant membrane stabilizer that is a precursor to acetylcholine.

ELASTIN FIBERS: protein fibers that, along with collagen, are responsible for the strength and texture of the skin.

EPIDERMIS: outer layer of the skin.

FIBROBLASTS: cells that produce collagen and elastin.

FLAVONOIDS: phytochemicals (plant-based chemicals) with strong antioxidant properties.

FREE RADICALS: unstable molecules that produce inflammation and promote aging.

GAMMA LINOLEIC ACID: essential fatty acid.

GLUTATHIONE PEROXIDASE: an enzyme that is essential for the removal of toxins produced by lipid metabolism.

GLYCATION: attachment of sugar to a protein. When it occurs to collagen fibers, it creates cross-linking that leads to loss of elasticity and decline in skin tone.

HGH (HUMAN GROWTH HORMONE): hormone secreted by the pituitary gland. Declining levels as we age are linked to weight gain, sagging skin, and lower energy levels.

HYDROXYL FREE RADICALS: particularly dangerous form of free radical.

HYDROXYTYROSOL: a polyphenol antioxidant found in Italian extra virgin olive oil.

HYPERTROPHIC SCAR: enlarged, raised scar that develops during healing.

INDOLES: powerful anticancer compounds found in cabbage, brussels sprouts, cauliflower, and kale.

INDUCIBLE NITRIC OXIDE: a metabolic end product that causes smooth muscle to relax.

KERATIN: the protein that is the primary constituent of hair, nails, and skin.

LEUKOTRIENE: compound produced by the arachidonic acid cascade that produces inflammatory changes throughout the body.

LYCOPENE: an antioxidant compound found in tomatoes.

MELANOCYTE: cell in the skin that produces and contains the pigment melanin.

NF-κB (NUCLEAR FACTOR KAPPAB): a transcription factor triggered by oxidative stress that in turn promotes production of highly inflammatory interleukins.

OLEIC ACID: a component of olive oil that helps omega-3 oil pass into the cell membrane.

OMEGA-3 FATTY ACID: Anti-inflammatory essential fatty acids found in fish, oatmeal, nuts, and soy products. Studies have shown that omega-3s can decrease risk of heart disease, several types of cancers, and relieve the pain of arthritis.

OXIDATIVE STRESS: a highly oxidized environment within cells where there is an excess of free radicals and a lack of antioxidants.

PHENYLBAUTYLNITRONE (PBN): a type of spin trap used to collect and detect free radicals.

PHOSPHATIDYL CHOLINE: found naturally in lecithin, it offers important protection to the cell plasma membrane.

POLYPHENOLS: antioxidant bioflavonoids found in tea and red wine.

PROANTHROCYANIDINS: strong antioxidants found in pine needles, grapes, and blueberries that boost antioxidant properties of vitamins E and C.

PROSTAGLANDINS: a group of inflammatory compounds derived from arachidonic acid.

QUERCETIN: polyphenol antioxidant found in red wine.

REDOX LEVEL: a ratio of free radicals to antioxidants in the cell.

ROSACEA: chronic inflammation of the skin on the nose, chin, and forehead, characterized by redness or acnelike eruptions.

SATURATED FAT: a fatty acid that increases risk for heart disease. Found primarily in animal fats such as butter and in beef and pork.

SECRETAGOGUE: compound that increases secretion from cells.

SPIN TRAPS: a technique for detecting free radicals in living organisms.

SUPEROXIDISMUTASE (SOD): antioxidant produced by the body in response presence of free radicals.

TETRONIC ACID: a compound with a molecular structure very similar to vitamin C that lightens and evens out irregular pigmentation of the skin.

TOCOPHEROL: a fraction of vitamin E that disarms free radicals.

TOCOTRIENOL: a fraction of vitamin E that has powerful antioxidant potential.

TRANSCRIPTION FACTORS: compounds made in the body that trigger genetic transcription process.

TUMOR NECROSIS FACTOR: an inflammatory compound that can inhibit tumor growth.

References

Chapter 1

Benton, D. The impact of the supply of glucose to the brain on mood and memory. *Nutr Rev.* 2001 Jan. 59(1 Pt 2): S20–1.

Dye, L., and J. E. Blundell. Menstrual cycle and appetite control: Implications for weight regulation. *Hum Reprod.* 1997 Jun. 12(6): 1142–1151.

Fernstrom, J. D. Carbohydrate ingestion and brain serotonin synthesis: Relevance to a putative control loop for regulating carbohydrate ingestion, and effects of aspartame consumption. *Appetite.* 1988, 11 Suppl 1: 35–41.

Leibenluft, E., P. L. Fiero, and D. R. Rubinow. Effects of the menstrual cycle on dependent variables in mood disorder research. *Arch Gen Psychiatry.* 1994 Oct.; 51(10): 761–781.

Wurtman, R. J., and J. J. Wurtman. Brain serotonin, carbohydrate-craving, obesity and depression. *Obes Res.* 1995 Nov.; 3 Suppl 4: 477S–480S.

———. Do carbohydrates affect food intake via neurotransmitter activity? *Appetite.* 1988; 11 Suppl 1: 42–47.

Chapter 2

Adler, V., Z. Yin, K. D. Tew, and Z. Ronai. Role of redox potential and reactive oxygen species in stress signaling. *Oncogene.* 1999, Nov. 1; 18(45): 6104–6111.

Brod, S. A. Unregulated inflammation shortens human functional longevity. *Inflamm Res.* 2000 Nov.; 49(11): 561–570.

Camhi, S. L., P. Lee, and A. M. Choi. The oxidative stress response. *New Horiz.* 1995 May; 3(2): 170–182.

Christman, J. W., T. S. Blackwell, and B. H. Juurlink. Redox regulation of nuclear factor kappa B: Therapeutic potential for attenuating inflammatory responses. *Brain Pathol.* 2000 Jan.; 10(1): 153–162.

Gius, D., A. Botero, S. Shah, and H. A. Curry. Intracellular oxidation/reduction status in the regulation of transcription factors NF-kappaB and AP-1. *Toxicol Lett.* 1999, Jun. 1; 106(2–3): 93–106.

Harman D. Aging and oxidative stress. *J Int Fed Clin Chem.* 1998 Mar.; 10(1): 24–27.

———. Extending functional life span. *Exp Gerontol.* 1998 Jan.–Mar.; 33(1–2): 95–112. Review.

Hedbom, E., and H. J. Hauselmann. Molecular aspects of pathogenesis in osteoarthritis: The role of inflammation. *Cell Mol Life Sci.* 2002 Jan.; 59(1): 45–53.

Hensley, K., K. A. Robinson, S. P. Gabbita, S. Salsman, and R. A. Floyd. Reactive oxygen species, cell signaling, and cell injury. *Free Radic Biol Med.* 2000, May 15; 28(10): 1456–1462.

Lavrovsky, Y., B. Chatterjee, R. A. Clark, and A. K. Roy. Role of redox-regulated transcription factors in inflammation, aging and age-related diseases. *Exp Gerontol.* 2000 Aug.; 35(5): 521–532.

Mulvihill, N. T., and J. B. Foley. Inflammation in acute coronary syndromes. *Heart.* 2002 Mar.; 87(3): 201–204.

Spiteller, G. Peroxidation of linoleic acid and its relation to aging and age dependent diseases. *Mech Ageing Dev.* 2001, May 31; 122(7): 617–657.

Terman, A. Garbage catastrophe theory of aging: Imperfect removal of oxidative damage? *Redox Rep.* 2001; 6(1): 15–26.

Wilhelm, J. Metabolic aspects of membrane lipid peroxidation. *Acta Univ Carol Med Monogr.* 1990; 137: 1–53.

Zs-Nagy, I. The membrane hypothesis of aging: Its relevance to recent progress in genetic research. *J Mol Med.* 1997 Oct.; 75(10): 703–714.

Zs-Nagy, I., and I. Semsei. Centrophenoxine increases the rates of total and mRNA synthesis in the brain cortex of old rats: An explanation of its action in terms of the membrane hypothesis of aging. *Exp Gerontol.* 1984; 19(3): 171–178.

Zs-Nagy, I., R. G. Cutler, and I. Semsei. Dysdifferentiation hypothesis of aging and cancer: A comparison with the membrane hypothesis of aging. *Ann NY Acad Sci.* 1988; 521: 215–225.

Chapter 3

Alarcon de la Lastra, C., M. D. Barranco, V. Motilva, and J. M. Herrerias. Mediterranean diet and health: Biological importance of olive oil. *Curr Pharm Des.* 2001 Jul.; 7(10): 933–950.

Alkadhi, K. A. Endplate channel actions of a hemicholinium-3 analog, DMAE. *Naunyn Schmiedebergs Arch Pharmacol.* 1986 Mar.; 332(3): 230–235.

Ascherio, A., M. J. Stampfer, and W. C. Willett. Transfatty acids and coronary heart disease. *Background and Scientific Review.* Departments of Nutrition and Epidemiology, Harvard School of Public Health; The Channing Laboratory, Department of Medicine, Brigham and Women's Hospital. http://www.hsph. harvard.edu/reviews/transfats.html

Cefalu, W. T., A. D. Bell-Farrow, Z. Q. Wang, W. E. Sonntag, M. X. Fu, J. W. Baynes, and S. R. Thorpe. Caloric restriction decreases age-dependent accumulation of the glycoxidation products, N epsilon-(carboxymethyl)lysine and pentosidine, in rat skin collagen. *J Gerontol A Biol Sci Med Sci.* 1995 Nov.; 50(6): B337–B341.

Clevidence, B. A., J. T. Judd, E. J. Schaefer, et al. Plasma lipoprotein (a) levels in men and women consuming diets enriched in saturated, Cis-, or Trans-monounsaturated fatty acids. *Arterioscler Thromb Vasc Biol.* 1997; 17: 1657–1661.

Cole, A. C., E. M. Gisoldi, and R. M. Grossman. Clinical and consumer evaluations of improved facial appearance after one month use of topical dimethyl-aminoethanol. Poster presentation, American Academy of Dermatology. 2002, Feb. 22–26; New Orleans, USA.

Das, U. N. Essential fatty acid metabolism in patients with essential hypertension, diabetes mellitus and coronary heart disease. *Prostaglandins Leukot Essent Fatty Acids.* 1995 Jun.; 52(6): 387–391.

———. GLUT-4, tumor necrosis factor, essential fatty acids and daf-genes and their role in insulin resistance and non-insulin dependent diabetes mellitus. Prostaglandins Leukot Essent Fatty Acids. 1999 Jan.; 60(1): 13–20.

de Lorgeril, M., and P. Salen. Mediterranean type of diet for the prevention of coronary heart disease: A global perspective from the seven countries study to the most recent dietary trials. *Int J Vitam Nutr Res.* 2001 May; 71(3): 166–172.

Carlson, E. C., and V. M. Monnier. Differential effects of type 2 (non-insulin-dependent) diabetes mellitus on pentosidine formation in skin and glomerular basement membrane. *Diabetologia.* 1993 Oct.; 36(10): 936–941.

Duan, W., and M. P. Mattson. Dietary restriction and 2-deoxyglucose administration improve behavioral outcome and reduce degeneration of dopaminergic neurons in models of Parkinson's disease. *J Neurosci Res.* 1999, Jul. 15; 57(2): 195–206.

Favero, A., M. Parpinel, and S. Franceschi. Diet and risk of breast cancer: Major findings from an Italian case control study. *Biomed Pharmacother* (France). 1998; 52(3): 109–115.

Fu, M. X., J. R. Requena, A. J. Jenkins, T. J. Lyons, J. W. Baynes, and S. R. Thorpe. The advanced glycation end-product, Ne-(carboxymethyl)lysine, is a product of both lipid peroxidation and glycoxidation reactions. *J Biol Chem.* 1996; 271: 9982–9986.

Gandini, S., H. Merzenich, C. Robertson, et al. Meta-analysis of studies on breast cancer risk and diet the role of fruit and vegetable consumption and the intake of associated micronutrients. *Eur J Cancer* (England). Mar. 2000; 36(5): 636–646.

Grossman, R. M., E. M. Gisoldi, and A. C. Cole. Long-term safety and efficacy evaluation of a new skin firming technology: Dimethylaminoethanol. Poster presentation, American Academy of Dermatology, 2002, Feb. 22–26; New Orleans, USA.

Guerci, B., P. Bohme, A. Kearney-Schwartz, F. Zannad, and P. Drouin. Endothelial dysfunction and type 2 diabetes. Part 2: altered endothelial function and the effects of treatments in type 2 diabetes mellitus. *Diabetes Metab.* 2001 Sep.; 27(4 Pt 1): 436–447.

Hayden, J. M., and P. D. Reaven. Cardiovascular disease in diabetes mellitus type 2: A potential role for novel cardiovascular risk factors. *Curr Opin Lipidol.* 2000 Oct.; 11(5): 519–528.

Holt, S. H., J. C. Miller, and P. Petocz. An insulin index of foods: The insulin demand generated by 1000-kj portions of common foods. *Am J Clin Nutr.* 1997 Nov.; 66(5): 1264–1276.

Hu, F. B., R. M. van Dam, and S. Liu. Diet and risk of type 2 diabetes: The role of types of fat and carbohydrate. *Diabetologia.* 2001 Jul.; 44(7): 805–817.

James, M. J., R. A. Gibson, and L. G. Cleland. Dietary polyunsaturated fatty acids and inflammatory mediator production. *Am J Clin Nutr.* 2000 Jan.; 71(1 Suppl): 343S–348S.

Lin, Y., M. W. Rajala, J. P. Berger, D. E. Moller, N. Barzilai, and P. E. Scherer. Hyperglycemia-induced production of acute phase reactants in adipose tissue. *J Biol Chem.* 2001, Nov. 9; 276(45): 42077–42083.

Lingelbach, L. B., A. E. Mitchell, R. B. Rucker, and R. B. McDonald. Accumulation of advanced glycation endproducts in aging male fischer 344 rats during long-term feeding of various dietary carbohydrates. *J Nutr.* 2000 May; 130(5): 1247–1255.

Liu, S., and J. E. Manson. Dietary carbohydrates, physical inactivity, obesity, and the "metabolic syndrome" as predictors of coronary heart disease. *Curr Opin Lipidol.* 2001 Aug.; 12(4): 395–404.

Martinez-Dominguez, E., R. de la Puerta, and V. Ruiz-Gutierrez. Protective effects upon experimental inflammation models of a polyphenol-supplemented virgin olive oil diet. *Inflamm Res.* 2001 Feb.; 50(2): 102–106.

McCarty, M. F. Nitric oxide deficiency, leukocyte activation, and resultant ischemia are crucial to the pathogenesis of diabetic retinopathy/neuropathy— preventive potential of antioxidants, essential fatty acids, chromium, ginkgolides, and pentoxifylline. *Med Hypotheses.* 1998 May; 50(5): 435–449.

McKeown, N. Antioxidants and breast cancer. *Nutr Rev* (U.S.). 1999 Oct., 57(10): 321–324.

Mensink, R. P., and M. B. Katan. Effect of dietary fatty acids on serum lipids and lipoproteins: A meta-analysis of 27 trials. *Arteriosclerosis and Thrombosis.* 1992; 12: 911–919.

Middleton, E. Jr., C. Kandaswami, and T. C. Theoharides. The effects of plant flavonoids on mammalian cells: Implications for inflammation, heart disease, and cancer. *Pharmacol Rev.* 2000 Dec.; 52(4): 673–751.

Miller, J. B., E. Pang, and L. Bramall. Rice: A high or low glycemic index food? *Am J Clin Nutr.* 1992 Dec.; 56(6): 1034–1036.

Niemela, O., S. Parkkila, M. Pasanen, Y. Iimuro, B. Bradford, and R. G. Thurman. Early alcoholic liver injury: Formation of protein adducts with acetaldehyde and lipid peroxidation products, and expression of CYP2E1 and CYP3A. *Alcohol Clin Exp Res.* 1998 Dec.; 22(9): 2118–2124.

Normand, S., Y. Khalfallah, C. Louche-Pelissier, C. Pachiaudi, J. M. Antoine, S. Blanc, M. Desage, J. P. Riou, and M. Laville. Influence of dietary fat on postprandial glucose metabolism (exogenous and endogenous) using intrinsically (13)C-enriched durum wheat. *Br J Nutr.* 2001 Jul.; 86(1): 3–11.

Owen, R. W., A. Giacosa, W. E. Hull, R. Haubner, G. Wurtele, B. Spiegelhalder, and H. R. Bartsch. Olive-oil consumption and health: The possible role of antioxidants. *Lancet Oncol.* 2000 Oct.; 1: 107–112.

Owen, R. W., A. Giacosa, W. E. Hull, R. Haubner, B. Spiegelhalder, and H. Bartsch. The antioxidant/anticancer potential of phenolic compounds isolated from olive oil. *Eur J Cancer.* 2000 Jun.; 36(10): 1235–1247.

Pawlak, D. B., J. M. Bryson, G. S. Denyer, and J. C. Brand-Miller. High glycemic index starch promotes hypersecretion of insulin and higher body fat in rats without affecting insulin sensitivity. *J Nutr.* 2001 Jan.; 131(1): 99–104.

Purba, M. B., A. Kouris-Blazos, N. Wattanapenpaiboon, W. Lukito, E. M. Rothenberg, B. C. Steen, and M. L. Wahlqvist. Skin wrinkling: Can food make a difference? *J Am Coll Nutr.* 2001 Feb.; 20(1): 71–80.

Radcliffe, J. D., and A. C. Glass. Dietary cottonseed protein can reduce the severity of retinoid-induced hypertriglyceridemia. *Cancer Detect Prev.* 1994; 18(5): 401–406.

Rittie, L., A. Berton, J. C. Monboisse, W. Hornebeck, and P. Gillery. Decreased contraction of glycated collagen lattices coincides with impaired matrix metalloproteinase production. *Biochem Biophys Res Commun.* 1999, Oct. 22; 264(2): 488–492.

Roman, R. J. P-450 metabolites of arachidonic acid in the control of cardiovascular function. *Physiol Rev.* 2002 Jan.; 82(1): 131–185.

Sell, D. R. Ageing promotes the increase of early glycation Amadori product as assessed by epsilon-N-(2-furoylmethyl)-L-lysine (furosine) levels in rodent skin collagen. The relationship to dietary restriction and glycoxidation. *Mech Ageing Dev.* 1997 Apr.; 95(1–2): 81–99.

Semsei, I., and I. Zs-Nagy. Superoxide radical scavenging ability of centrophenoxine and its salt dependence in vitro. *J Free Radic Biol Med.* 1985; 1(5–6): 403–408.

Simopoulos, A. P. Essential fatty acids in health and chronic disease. *Am J Clin Nutr.* 1999 Sep.; 70(3 Suppl): 560S–569S.

Stoll, B. A. Essential fatty acids, insulin resistance, and breast cancer risk. *Nutr Cancer.* 1998; 31(1): 72–77.

Trichopoulou, A., P. Lagiou, H. Kuper, and D. Trichopoulos. Cancer and Mediterranean dietary traditions. *Cancer Epidemiol Biomarkers Prev.* 2000 Sep.; 9(9): 869–873.

USDA Nutrient Database for Standard Reference, Release 14. http://www.nal.usda.gov/fnic/foodcomp/Data/SR14/reports/sr14page.htm

Visioli, F., L. Borsani, and C. Galli. Diet and prevention of coronary heart disease: The potential role of phytochemicals. *Cardiovasc Res* (Netherlands), 2000, Aug. 18; 47(3): 419–425.

Visioli, F., C. Galli, E. Plasmati, S. Viappiani, A. Hernandez, C. Colombo, and A. Sala. Olive phenol hydroxytyrosol prevents passive smoking-induced oxidative stress. *Circulation.* 2000, Oct. 31; 102(18): 2169–2171.

Wallenfeldt, K., J. Hulthe, L. Bokemark, J. Wikstrand, and B. Fagerberg. Carotid and femoral atherosclerosis, cardiovascular risk factors and C-reactive protein in relation to smokeless tobacco use or smoking in 58-year-old men. *J Intern Med.* 2001 Dec.; 250(6): 492–501.

Willett, W. C. *Eat, drink, and be healthy: The Harvard Medical School Guide to healthy eating.* New York: Simon & Schuster Source, 2001.

Yim, M. B., H. S. Yim, C. Lee, S. O. Kang, and P. B. Chock. Protein glycation: Creation of catalytic sites for free radical generation. *Ann NY Acad Sci.* 2001 Apr.; 928: 48–53.

Yu, M. J., et al. Phenothiazines as lipid peroxidation inhibitors and cytoprotective agents. *J Med Chem.* 1992, Feb. 21; 35(4): 716–724.

Zammit, V. A., I. J. Waterman, D. Topping, and G. McKay. Insulin stimulation of hepatic triacylglycerol secretion and the etiology of insulin resistance. *J Nutr.* 2001 Aug.; 131(8): 2074–2077.

Ziboh, V. A., C. C. Miller, and Y. Cho. Metabolism of polyunsaturated fatty acids by skin epidermal enzymes: Generation of anti-inflammatory and antiproliferative metabolites. *Am J Clin Nutr.* 2000 Jan.; 71(1 Suppl): 361S–366S.

Zs-Nagy I. On the role of intracellular physicochemistry in quantitative gene expression during aging and the effect of centrophenoxine: A review. *Arch Gerontol Geriatr.* 1989 Nov.–Dec.; 9(3): 215–229.

Zs-Nagy, I., and I. Semsei. Centrophenoxine increases the rates of total and mRNA synthesis in the brain cortex of old rats: An explanation of its action in terms of the membrane hypothesis of aging. *Exp Gerontol.* 1984; 19(3): 171–178.

Chapter 4 (general)

Berbis P., S. Hesse, and Y. Privat. Essential fatty acids and the skin. *Allerg Immunol* (Paris). 1990 Jun.; 22(6): 225–231.

Berdanier, C. D. *Advanced nutrition: micronutrients.* Boca Raton: CRC Press, January 15, 1998.

———. *CRC desk reference for nutrition.* Boca Raton: CRC Press, January 15, 1997.

Bierhaus, A., et al. Advanced glycation end product-induced activation of NF-kappaB is suppressed by alpha-lipoic acid in cultured endothelial cells. *Diabetes.* 1997 Sep.; 46(9): 1481–1490.

Bissett, D. L., R. Chatterjee, and D. P. Hannon. Photoprotective effect of superoxide-scavenging antioxidants against ultraviolet radiation-induced chronic skin damage in the hairless mouse. *Photodermatol Photoimmunol Photomed.* 1990 Apr.; 7(2): 56–62.

Council for Responsible Nutrition. Safety of Vitamins and Minerals. Washington: Feb. 2, 2002. http://www.crnusa.org/Shellscireg000001.html

Curcuma longa (turmeric). Monograph. *Altern Med Rev.* 2001 Sep.; (6 Suppl): S62–S66.

Food and Nutrition Board, Institute of Medicine. *Dietary reference intakes: A risk assessment model for establishing upper intake levels for nutrients.* Washington: National Academy Press, 1999.

Fuchs, J., and R. Milbradt. Antioxidant inhibition of skin inflammation induced by reactive oxidants: Evaluation of the redox couple dihydrolipoate/lipoate. *Skin Pharmacol.* 1994; 7(5): 278–284.

Gismondo, M. R., L. Drago, M. C. Fassina, I. Vaghi, R. Abbiati, and E. Grossi. Immunostimulating effect of oral glutamine. *Dig Dis Sci* 1998 Aug.; 43(8): 1752–1754.

Grimble, R. F. Nutritional modulation of immune function. *Proc Nutr Soc.* 2001 Aug.; 60(3): 389–397.

Hagen, T. M., J. Liu, J. Lykkesfeldt, C. M. Wehr, R. T. Ingersoll, V. Vinarsky, J. C. Bartholomew, and B. N. Ames. Feeding acetyl-L-carnitine and lipoic acid to old rats significantly improves metabolic function while decreasing oxidative stress. *Proc Natl Acad Sci USA.* 2002, Feb. 19; 99(4): 1870–1875.

Han, D., G. Handelman, L. Marcocci, C. K. Sen, S. Roy, H. Kobuchi, H. J. Tritschler, L. Flohe, and L. Packer. Lipoic acid increases de novo synthesis of cellular glutathione by improving cystine utilization. *Biofactors.* 1997; 6(3): 321–338.

Isseroff, R. R. Fish again for dinner! The role of fish and other dietary oils in the therapy of skin disease. *J Am Acad Dermatol.* 1988 Dec.; 19(6): 1073–1080.

Johnston, C. S., and B. Luo. Comparison of the absorption and excretion of three commercially available sources of vitamin C. *J Am Diet Assoc.* 1994 Jul.; 94(7): 779–781.

Kagan, V. E., A. Shvedova, E. Serbinova, S. Khan, C. Swanson, R. Powell, and L. Packer. Dihydrolipoic acid—A universal antioxidant both in the membrane and in the aqueous phase. Reduction of peroxyl, ascorbyl and chromanoxyl radicals. *Biochem Pharmacol.* 1992, Oct. 20; 44(8): 1637–1649.

Kunt, T., et al. Alpha-lipoic acid reduces expression of vascular cell adhesion molecule-1 and endothelial adhesion of human monocytes after stimulation with advanced glycation end products. *Clin Sci* (London). 1999 Jan.; 96(1): 75–82.

Lim, G. P., T. Chu, F. Yang, W. Beech, S. A. Frautschy, and G. M. Cole. The curry spice curcumin reduces oxidative damage and amyloid pathology in an Alzheimer transgenic mouse. *J Neurosci.* 2001, Nov. 1; 21(21): 8370–8377.

Liu, J., E. Head, A. M. Gharib, W. Yuan, R. T. Ingersoll, T. M. Hagen, C. W. Cotman, and B. N. Ames. Memory loss in old rats is associated with brain mitochondrial decay and RNA/DNA oxidation: Partial reversal by feeding acetyl-L-carnitine and/or R-alpha-lipoic acid. *Proc Natl Acad Sci USA.* 2002, Feb. 19; 99(4): 2356–2361.

Liu, J., D. W. Killilea, and B. N. Ames. Age-associated mitochondrial oxidative decay: Improvement of carnitine acetyltransferase substrate-binding affinity and activity in brain by feeding old rats acetyl-L-carnitine and/or R-alpha-lipoic acid. *Proc Natl Acad Sci USA.* 2002, Feb. 19; 99(4): 1876–1881.

Melhem, M. F., P. A. Craven, J. Liachenko, and F. R. DeRubertis. Alpha-lipoic acid attenuates hyperglycemia and prevents glomerular mesangial matrix expansion in diabetes. *J Am Soc Nephrol.* 2002 Jan.; 13(1): 108–116.

Nair, S., R. Nagar, and R. Gupta. Antioxidant phenolics and flavonoids in common Indian foods. *J Assoc Physicians India.* 1998 Aug.; 46(8): 708–710.

Packer, L., E. H. Witt, and H. J. Tritschler. Alpha-lipoic acid as a biological antioxidant. *Free Radic Biol Med.* 1995 Aug.; 19(2): 227–250.

Panel on Dietary Antioxidants and Related Compounds, Subcommittees on Upper Reference Levels of Nutrients and Interpretation and Uses of DRIs, and the Standing Committee on the Scientific Evaluation of Dietary Reference Intakes, Food and Nutrition Board. *Dietary Reference Intakes for Vitamin C, Vitamin E, Selenium, and Carotenoids.* Washington: National Academy Press, 2000.

Panel on Micronutrients, Subcommittees on Upper Reference Levels of Nutrients and of Interpretation and Use of Dietary Reference Intakes, and the Standing Committee on the Scientific Evaluation of Dietary Reference Intakes, Food and Nutrition Board, Institute of Medicine. *Dietary Reference Intakes for Vitamin A, Vitamin K, Arsenic, Boron, Chromium, Copper, Iodine, Iron, Manganese, Molybdenum, Nickel, Silicon, Vanadium, and Zinc.* Washington: National Academy Press, 2001.

Perricone, N., K. Nagy, F. Horvath, G. Dajko, I. Uray, and I. Zs-Nagy. Alpha lipoic acid (ALA) protects proteins against the hydroxyl free radical-induced alterations: Rationale for its geriatric application. *Arch Gerontol Geriatr.* 1999 Jul.–Aug.; 29 (1): 45–56.

Perricone, N. V. Topical 5% alpha lipoic acid cream in the treatment of cutaneous rhytids. *Aesthetic Surgery Journal.* 2000 May/Jun.; 20 (3): 218–222.

Podda, M., M. Rallis, M. G. Traber, L. Packer, and H. I. Maibach. Kinetic study of cutaneous and subcutaneous distribution following topical application of [7,8–14C]rac-alpha-lipoic acid onto hairless mice. *Biochem Pharmacol.* 1996, Aug. 23; 52(4): 627–633.

Podda, M., H. J. Tritschler, H. Ulrich, and L. Packer. Alpha-lipoic acid supplementation prevents symptoms of vitamin E deficiency. *Biochem Biophys Res Commun.* 1994, Oct. 14; 204(1): 98–104.

Podda, M., T. M., Zollner, M. Grundmann-Kollmann, J. J. Thiele, L. Packer, and R. Kaufmann. Activity of alpha-lipoic acid in the protection against oxidative stress in skin. *Curr Probl Dermatol.* 2001; 29: 43–51.

Prendiville, J. S., and L. N. Manfredi. Skin signs of nutritional disorders. *Semin Dermatol.* 1992 Mar.; 11(1): 88–97.

Standing Committee on the Scientific Evaluation of Dietary Reference Intakes and its Panel on Folate, Other B Vitamins, and Choline and Subcommittee on Upper Reference Levels of Nutrients, Food and Nutrition Board, Institute of Medicine. *Dietary Reference Intakes for Thiamin, Riboflavin, Niacin, Vitamin B6, Folate, Vitamin B12, Pantothenic Acid, Biotin, and Choline.* Washington: National Academy Press, 2000.

Standing Committee on the Scientific Evaluation of Dietary Reference Intakes,

Food and Nutrition Board, Institute of Medicine. *Dietary Reference Intakes: Proposed Definition and Plan for Review of Dietary Antioxidants and Related Compounds.* Washington: National Academy Press, 1998.

———. *Dietary Reference Intakes for Calcium, Phosphorus, Magnesium, Vitamin D, and Fluoride.* Washington: National Academy Press, 1997.

Subcommittees on Interpretation and Uses of Dietary Reference Intakes and Upper Reference Levels of Nutrients, and the Standing Committee on the Scientific Evaluation of Dietary Reference Intakes, Food and Nutrition Board, Institute of Medicine. *Dietary Reference Intakes: Applications in Dietary Assessment.* Washington: National Academy Press, 2001.

Subcommittee on the Tenth Edition of the Recommended Dietary Allowances, Food and Nutrition Board, Commission on Life Sciences, National Research Council. *Recommended Dietary Allowances: 10th Edition.* Washington: National Academy Press, 1989.

Ziboh, V. A., and C. C. Miller. Essential fatty acids and polyunsaturated fatty acids: Significance in cutaneous biology. *Annu Rev Nutr.* 1990; 10: 433–450.

Ziboh, V. A., C. C. Miller, and Y. Cho. Metabolism of polyunsaturated fatty acids by skin epidermal enzymes: Generation of anti-inflammatory and antiproliferative metabolites. *Am J Clin Nutr.* 2000 Jan.; 71(1 Suppl): 361S–366S.

Chapter 4 (by subtopic)

EFAs

Berbis, P., S. Hesse, and Y. Privat. Essential fatty acids and the skin. *Allerg Immunol* (Paris). 1990 Jun.; 22(6): 225–231.

Isseroff, R. R. Fish again for dinner! The role of fish and other dietary oils in the therapy of skin disease. *J Am Acad Dermatol.* 1988 Dec.; 19(6): 1073–1080.

Prendiville, J. S., and L. N. Manfredi. Skin signs of nutritional disorders. *Semin Dermatol.* 1992 Mar.; 11(1): 88–97.

Ziboh, V. A., and C. C. Miller. Essential fatty acids and polyunsaturated fatty acids: Significance in cutaneous biology. *Annu Rev Nutr.* 1990; 10: 433–450.

Ziboh, V. A., C. C. Miller, and Y. Cho. Metabolism of polyunsaturated fatty acids by skin epidermal enzymes: Generation of anti-inflammatory and antiproliferative metabolites. *Am J Clin Nutr.* 2000 Jan.; 71(1 Suppl): 361S–366S.

RDIs, NOAELs, Vitamin and Mineral properties

Berdanier, C. D. *Advanced Nutrition: Micronutrients.* Boca Raton: CRC Press, January 15, 1998.

———. *CRC Desk Reference for Nutrition.* Boca Raton: CRC Press, January 15, 1997.

Council for Responsible Nutrition. Safety of Vitamins and Minerals. Washington: Feb. 2, 2002. http://www.crnusa.org/Shellscireg000001.html

Food and Nutrition Board, Institute of Medicine. *Dietary Reference Intakes: A Risk*

Assessment Model for Establishing Upper Intake Levels for Nutrients. Washington: National Academy Press, 1999.

Panel on Dietary Antioxidants and Related Compounds, Subcommittees on Upper Reference Levels of Nutrients and Interpretation and Uses of DRIs, Standing Committee on the Scientific Evaluation of Dietary Reference Intakes, Food and Nutrition Board. *Dietary Reference Intakes for Vitamin C, Vitamin E, Selenium, and Carotenoids.* Washington: National Academy Press, 2000.

Panel on Micronutrients, Subcommittees on Upper Reference Levels of Nutrients and of Interpretation and Use of Dietary Reference Intakes, and the Standing Committee on the Scientific Evaluation of Dietary Reference Intakes, Food and Nutrition Board, Institute of Medicine. *Dietary Reference Intakes for Vitamin A, Vitamin K, Arsenic, Boron, Chromium, Copper, Iodine, Iron, Manganese, Molybdenum, Nickel, Silicon, Vanadium, and Zinc.* Washington: National Academy Press, 2001.

Standing Committee on the Scientific Evaluation of Dietary Reference Intakes, Food and Nutrition Board, Institute of Medicine. *Dietary Reference Intakes: Proposed Definition and Plan for Review of Dietary Antioxidants and Related Compounds.* Washington: National Academy Press, 1998.

———. *Dietary Reference Intakes for Calcium, Phosphorus, Magnesium, Vitamin D, and Fluoride.* Washington: National Academy Press, 1997.

Standing Committee on the Scientific Evaluation of Dietary Reference Intakes and its Panel on Folate, Other B Vitamins, and Choline and Subcommittee on Upper Reference Levels of Nutrients, Food and Nutrition Board, Institute of Medicine. *Dietary Reference Intakes for Thiamin, Riboflavin, Niacin, Vitamin B6, Folate, Vitamin B12, Pantothenic Acid, Biotin, and Choline.* Washington: National Academy Press, 2000.

Subcommittees on Interpretation and Uses of Dietary Reference Intakes and Upper Reference Levels of Nutrients, and the Standing Committee on the Scientific Evaluation of Dietary Reference Intakes, Food and Nutrition Board, Institute of Medicine. *Dietary Reference Intakes: Applications in Dietary Assessment.* Washington: National Academy Press, 2001.

Subcommittee on the Tenth Edition of the Recommended Dietary Allowances, Food and Nutrition Board, Commission on Life Sciences, National Research Council. *Recommended Dietary Allowances: 10th Edition.* Washington: National Academy Press, 1989.

ALA

Bierhaus, A., et al. Advanced glycation end product-induced activation of NF-kappaB is suppressed by alpha-lipoic acid in cultured endothelial cells. *Diabetes.* 1997 Sep.; 46(9): 1481–1490.

Fuchs, J., and R. Milbradt. Antioxidant inhibition of skin inflammation induced by reactive oxidants: Evaluation of the redox couple dihydrolipoate/lipoate. *Skin Pharmacol.* 1994; 7(5): 278–284.

Han, D., G. Handelman, L. Marcocci, C. K. Sen, S. Roy, H. Kobuchi, H. J.

Tritschler, L. Flohe, and L. Packer. Lipoic acid increases de novo synthesis of cellular glutathione by improving cystine utilization. *Biofactors.* 1997; 6(3): 321–338.

Kagan, V. E., A. Shvedova, E. Serbinova, S. Khan, C. Swanson, R. Powell, and L. Packer. Dihydrolipoic acid—A universal antioxidant both in the membrane and in the aqueous phase. Reduction of peroxyl, ascorbyl and chromanoxyl radicals. *Biochem Pharmacol.* 1992, Oct. 20; 44(8): 1637–1649.

Kunt, T., et al. Alpha-lipoic acid reduces expression of vascular cell adhesion molecule-1 and endothelial adhesion of human monocytes after stimulation with advanced glycation end products. *Clin Sci* (London). 1999 Jan.; 96(1): 75–82.

Melhem, M. F., P. A. Craven, J. Liachenko, and F. R. DeRubertis. Alpha-lipoic acid attenuates hyperglycemia and prevents glomerular mesangial matrix expansion in diabetes. *J Am Soc Nephrol.* 2002 Jan.; 13(1): 108–116.

Packer, L., E. H. Witt, and H. J. Tritschler. Alpha-lipoic acid as a biological antioxidant. *Free Radic Biol Med.* 1995 Aug.; 19(2): 227–250.

Perricone, N., K. Nagy, F. Horvath, G. Dajko, I. Uray, and I. Zs-Nagy. Alpha lipoic acid (ALA) protects proteins against the hydroxyl free radical-induced alterations: Rationale for its geriatric application. *Arch Gerontol Geriatr.* 1999 Jul.–Aug.; 29(1): 45–56.

Perricone, N. V. Topical 5% alpha lipoic acid cream in the treatment of cutaneous rhytids. *Aesthetic Surgery Journal.* 2000 May/June; 20(3): 218–222.

Podda, M., M. Rallis, M. G. Traber, L. Packer, and H. I. Maibach. Kinetic study of cutaneous and subcutaneous distribution following topical application of [7,8-14C]rac-alpha-lipoic acid onto hairless mice. *Biochem Pharmacol.* 1996, Aug. 23; 52(4): 627–633.

Podda, M., H. J. Tritschler, H. Ulrich, and L. Packer. Alpha-lipoic acid supplementation prevents symptoms of vitamin E deficiency. *Biochem Biophys Res Commun.* 1994, Oct. 14; 204(1): 98–104.

Podda, M., T. M. Zollner, M. Grundmann-Kollmann, J. J. Thiele, L. Packer, and R. Kaufmann. Activity of alpha-lipoic acid in the protection against oxidative stress in skin. *Curr Probl Dermatol.* 2001; 29: 43–51.

Vitamin C

Bissett, D. L., R. Chatterjee, and D. P. Hannon. Photoprotective effect of superoxide-scavenging antioxidants against ultraviolet radiation-induced chronic skin damage in the hairless mouse. *Photodermatol Photoimmunol Photomed.* 1990 Apr.; 7(2): 56–62.

Ester C

Johnston, C. S., and B. Luo. Comparison of the absorption and excretion of three commercially available sources of vitamin C. *J Am Diet Assoc.* 1994 Jul.; 94(7): 779–781.

TURMERIC

Curcuma longa (turmeric), monograph. *Altern Med Rev.* 2001 Sep.; 6 Suppl: S62–S66.

Lim, G. P., T. Chu, F. Yang, W. Beech, S. A. Frautschy, and G. M. Cole. The curry spice curcumin reduces oxidative damage and amyloid pathology in an Alzheimer transgenic mouse. *J Neurosci.* 2001, Nov. 1; 21(21): 8370–8377.

Nair, S., R. Nagar, and R. Gupta. Antioxidant phenolics and flavonoids in common Indian foods. *J Assoc Physicians India.* 1998 Aug.; 46(8): 708–710.

ACETYL L-CARNITINE

Hagen, T. M., J. Liu, J. Lykkesfeldt, C. M. Wehr, R. T. Ingersoll, V. Vinarsky, J. C. Bartholomew, and B. N. Ames. Feeding acetyl-L-carnitine and lipoic acid to old rats significantly improves metabolic function while decreasing oxidative stress. *Proc Natl Acad Sci USA.* 2002, Feb. 19; 99(4): 1870–1875.

Liu, J., E. Head, A. M. Gharib, W. Yuan, R. T. Ingersoll, T. M. Hagen, C. W. Cotman, and B. N. Ames. Memory loss in old rats is associated with brain mitochondrial decay and RNA/DNA oxidation: Partial reversal by feeding acetyl-L-carnitine and/or R-alpha-lipoic acid. *Proc Natl Acad Sci USA.* 2002, Feb. 19; 99(4): 2356–2361.

Liu, J., D. W. Killilea, and B. N. Ames. Age-associated mitochondrial oxidative decay: Improvement of carnitine acetyltransferase substrate-binding affinity and activity in brain by feeding old rats acetyl-L-carnitine and/or R-alpha-lipoic acid. *Proc Natl Acad Sci USA.* 2002, Feb. 19; 99(4): 1876–1881.

GLUTAMINE

M. R. Gismondo, L. Drago, M. C. Fassina, I. Vaghi, R. Abbiati, and E. Grossi. Immunostimulating effect of oral glutamine. *Dig Dis Sci.* 1998 Aug.; 43(8): 1752–1754.

Grimble, R. F. Nutritional modulation of immune function. *Proc Nutr Soc.* 2001 Aug.; 60(3): 389–397.

Chapter 5 (general)

Aleynik, S. I., M. A. Leo, M. K. Aleynik, and C. S. Lieber. Alcohol-induced pancreatic oxidative stress: Protection by phospholipid repletion. *Free Radic Biol Med.* 1999 Mar.; 26(5–6): 609–619.

Aleynik, S. I., M. A. Leo, X. Ma., M. K. Aleynik, and C. S. Lieber. Polyenylphosphatidylcholine prevents carbon tetrachloride-induced lipid peroxidation while it attenuates liver fibrosis. *J Hepatol.* 1997 Sep.; 27(3): 554–561.

Aleynik, S. I., M. A. Leo, U. Takeshige, M. K. Aleynik, and C. S. Lieber. Dilinoleoylphosphatidylcholine is the active antioxidant of polyenylphosphatidylcholine. *J Investig Med.* 1999 Nov.; 47(9): 507–512.

Alkadhi, K. A. Endplate channel actions of a hemicholinium-3 analog, DMAE. *Naunyn Schmiedebergs Arch Pharmacol.* 1986 Mar.; 332(3): 230–235.

Alvaro, D., A. Cantafora, C. Gandin, R. Masella, M. T. Santini, and M. Angelico. Selective hepatic enrichment of polyunsaturated phosphatidylcholines after intravenous administration of dimethylethanolamine in the rat. *Biochem Biophys Acta.* 1989, Nov. 6; 1006(1): 116–120.

Bierhaus, A., et al. Advanced glycation end product-induced activation of NF-kappaB is suppressed by alpha-lipoic acid in cultured endothelial cells. *Diabetes.* 1997 Sep.; 46(9): 1481–1490.

Bissett, D. L., R. Chatterjee, and D. P. Hannon. Photoprotective effect of superoxide-scavenging antioxidants against ultraviolet radiation-induced chronic skin damage in the hairless mouse. *Photodermatol Photoimmunol Photomed.* 1990 Apr.; 7(2): 56–62.

Briante, R., F. La Cara, M. P. Tonziello, F. Febbraio, and R. Nucci. Antioxidant activity of the main bioactive derivatives from oleuropein hydrolysis by hyperthermophilic beta-glycosidase. *J Agric Food Chem.* 2001 Jul.; 49(7): 3198–3203.

Cole, A. C., E. M. Gisoldi, and R. M. Grossman. Clinical and consumer evaluations of improved facial appearance after 1 month use of topical dimethylaminoethanol. Poster presentation, American Academy of Dermatology, 2002, Feb. 22–26; New Orleans, USA.

D'Angelo, S., C. Manna, V. Migliardi, O. Mazzoni, P. Morrica, G. Capasso, G. Pontoni, P. Galletti, and V. Zappia. Pharmacokinetics and metabolism of hydroxytyrosol, a natural antioxidant from olive oil. *Drug Metab Dispos.* 2001 Nov.; 29(11): 1492–1498.

de la Puerta, R., M. E. Martinez Dominguez, V. Ruiz-Gutierrez, J. A. Flavill, and J. R. Hoult. Effects of virgin olive oil phenolics on scavenging of reactive nitrogen species and upon nitrergic neurotransmission. *Life Sci.* 2001, Jul. 27; 69(10): 1213–1222.

Fuchs, J., and R. Milbradt. Antioxidant inhibition of skin inflammation induced by reactive oxidants: Evaluation of the redox couple dihydrolipoate/lipoate. *Skin Pharmacol.* 1994; 7(5): 278–284.

Fuchs, J., L. Packer, and G. Zimmer. *Lipoic Acid in Health and Disease.* New York: Marcel Dekker, 1997.

Genecov, D. G., K. E. Salyer, M. A. Kemer, S. Goldberg, J. Cho, and the International Society of Cleft Lip and Palate. Alpha lipoic acid (ALA) and scar formation in repaired cleft lips. 2001 Jun.; (462): 495–499.

Gordon, M. H., F. Paiva-Martins, and M. Almeida. Antioxidant activity of hydroxytyrosol acetate compared with that of other olive oil polyphenols. *J Agric Food Chem.* 2001 May; 49(5): 2480–2485.

Grossman, R. M., E. M. Gisoldi, and A. C. Cole. Long term safety and efficacy evaluation of a new skin firming technology: Dimethylaminoethanol. Poster presentation, American Academy of Dermatology, 2002, Feb. 22–26; New Orleans, USA.

Guyton, A. C. "Contraction of Skeletal Muscle," ch. 11 in *Textbook of Medical Physiology;* pp. 131–147. Philadelphia: W. B. Saunders Co., 1971.

Kagan, V. E., A. Shvedova, E. Serbinova, S. Khan, C. Swanson, R. Powell, and L. Packer. Dihydrolipoic acid—A universal antioxidant both in the membrane and in the aqueous phase. Reduction of peroxyl, ascorbyl and chromanoxyl radicals. *Biochem Pharmacol.* 1992, Oct. 20; 44(8): 1637–1649.

Kunt, T., et al. Alpha-lipoic acid reduces expression of vascular cell adhesion molecule-1 and endothelial adhesion of human monocytes after stimulation with advanced glycation end products. *Clin Sci* (London). 1999 Jan.; 96(1): 75–82.

Lichtenberger, L. M., J. J. Romero, W. M. de Ruijter, F. Behbod, R. Darling, A. Q. Ashraf, and S. K. Sanduja. Phosphatidylcholine association increases the anti-inflammatory and analgesic activity of ibuprofen in acute and chronic rodent models of joint inflammation: Relationship to alterations in bioavailability and cyclooxygenase-inhibitory potency. *J Pharmacol Exp Ther.* 2001 Jul.; 298(1): 279–287.

Meyer, M., H. L. Pahl, and P. A. Baeuerle. Regulation of the transcription factors NF-kappa B and AP-1 by redox changes. *Chem Biol Interact.* 1994 Jun.; 91(2–3): 91–100.

Meyer, M., R. Schreck, and P. A. Baeuerle. H_2O_2 and antioxidants have opposite effects on activation of NF-kappa B and AP-1 in intact cells: AP-1 as secondary antioxidant-responsive factor. *EMBO J.* 1993 May; 12(5): 2005–2015.

Nagy, I., and R. A. Floyd. Electron spin resonance spectroscopic demonstration of the hydroxyl free radical scavenger properties of dimethylaminoethanol in spin trapping experiments confirming the molecular basis for the biological effects of centrophenoxine. *Arch Gerontol Geriatr.* 1984 Dec.; 3(4): 297–310.

Nagy, I., and K. Nagy. On the role of cross-linking of cellular proteins in aging. *Mech Ageing Dev.* 1980 Sep.–Oct.; 14(1–2): 245–251.

Packer, L., S. Roy, and C. K. Sen. A-Lipoic acid: A metabolic antioxidant and potential redox modulator of transcription. *Advances in Pharmacology.* 1996; 38: 79–101.

Perricone, N., K. Nagy, F. Horvath, G. Dajko, I. Uray, and I. Zs-Nagy. The hydroxyl free radical reactions of ascorbyl palmitate as measured in various in vitro models. *Biochem Biophys Res Commun.* 1999, Sep. 7; 262(3): 661–665.

Perricone, N. V. Photoprotective and anti-inflammatory effects of topical ascorbyl palmitate. *J Geriatr Dermatol.* 1993; 1(1): 5–10.

———. Topical vitamin C ester (ascorbyl palmitate). Adapted from the first annual symposium on aging skin, San Diego, CA, February 21–23, 1997. *J Geriatric Dermatol.* 1997; 5(4): 162–170.

———. Topical vitamin C ester (ascorbyl palmitate). *J Geriatr Dermatol.* 1997; 5(4): 162–170.

———. Treatment of psoriasis with topical ascorbyl palmitate. *Clinical Research.* 1991; 39: 535A.

Rosenblat, G., et al. Acylated ascorbate stimulates collagen synthesis in cultured human foreskin fibroblasts at lower doses than does ascorbic acid. *Connect Tissue Res.* 1998; 37(3–4): 303–311.

Saliou, C., M. Kitazawa, L. McLaughlin, J. P. Yang, J. K. Lodge, T. Tetsuka, K. Iwasaki, J. Cillard, T. Okamoto, and L. Packer. Antioxidants modulate acute solar ultraviolet radiation-induced NF-kappa-B activation in a human keratinocyte cell line. *Free Radic Biol Med.* 1999 Jan.; 26(1–2): 174–183.

Semsei, I., and I. Zs-Nagy. Superoxide radical scavenging ability of centrophenoxine and its salt dependence in vitro. *J Free Radic Biol Med.* 1985; 1(5–6): 403–408.

Sen, C. K., and L. Packer. Antioxidant and redox regulation of gene transcription. *FASEB J.* 1996; 10: 709–720.

Serbinova, E., V. Kagan, D. Han, and L. Packer. Free radical recycling and intramembrane mobility in the antioxidant properties of alpha-tocopherol and alpha-tocotrienol. *Free Radic Biol Med.* 1991; 10(5): 263–275.

Serbinova, E. A., and L. Packer. Antioxidant properties of alpha-tocopherol and alpha-tocotrienol. *Methods Enzymol.* 1994; 234: 354–366.

Smart, R. C., and C. L. Crawford. Effect of ascorbic acid and its synthetic lipophilic derivative ascorbyl palmitate on phorbol ester-induced skin-tumor promotion in mice. *Am J Clin Nutr.* 1991 Dec.; 54(6 Suppl): 1266S–1273S.

Stryer, L. *Biochemistry, 3rd Edition.* San Francisco: W. H. Freeman and Co., 1988.

Suzuki, Y. J., B. B. Aggarwal, and L. Packer. Alpha-lipoic acid is a potent inhibitor of NF-kappa B activation in human T cells. *Biochem Biophys Res Commun.* 1992, Dec. 30; 189(3): 1709–1715.

Suzuki, Y. J., M. Mizuno, H. J. Tritschler, and L. Packer. Redox regulation of NF-kappa B DNA binding activity by dihydrolipoate. *Biochem Mol Biol Int.* 1995 Jun.; 36(2): 241–246.

Tebbe, B., S. Wu, C. C. Geilen, J. Eberle, V. Kodelja, and C. E. Orfanos. L-ascorbic acid inhibits UVA-induced lipid peroxidation and secretion of IL-1 alpha and IL-6 in cultured human keratinocytes in vitro. *J Invest Dermatol.* 1997 Mar.; 108(3): 302–306.

Thiele, J. J., M. G. Traber, and L. Packer. Depletion of human stratum corneum vitamin E: An early and sensitive in vivo marker of UV induced photooxidation. *J Invest Dermatol.* 1998 May; 110(5): 756–761.

Traber, M. G., M. Rallis, M. Podda, C. Weber, H. I. Maibach, and L. Packer. Penetration and distribution of alpha-tocopherol, alpha- or gamma-tocotrienols applied individually onto murine skin. *Lipids.* 1998 Jan.; 33(1): 87–91.

Traber, M. G., et al. Diet derived topically applied tocotrienols accumulate in skin and protect the tissue against UV light-induced oxidative stress. *Asia Pacific Journal of Clinical Nutrition.* 1997; 6: 63–67.

Tuck, K. L., M. P. Freeman, P. J. Hayball, G. L. Stretch, and I. Stupans. The in vivo fate of hydroxytyrosol and tyrosol, antioxidant phenolic constituents of olive oil, after intravenous and oral dosing of labeled compounds to rats. *J Nutr.* 2001 Jul.; 131(7): 1993–1996.

Visioli, F., A. Poli, and C. Gall. Antioxidant and other biological activities of phenols from olives and olive oil. *Med Res Rev.* 2002 Jan.; 22(1): 65–75.

Yu, M. J., et al. Phenothiazines as lipid peroxidation inhibitors and cytoprotective agents. *J Med Chem.* 1992, Feb. 21; 35(4): 716–724.

Zs-Nagy, I. On the role of intracellular physicochemistry in quantitative gene expression during aging and the effect of centrophenoxine. *Arch Gerontol Geriatr.* 1989 Nov.–Dec.; 9(3): 215–229.

Zs-Nagy, I., and I. Semsei. Centrophenoxine increases the rates of total and mRNA synthesis in the brain cortex of old rats: An explanation of its action in terms of the membrane hypothesis of aging. *Exp Gerontol.* 1984; 19(3): 171–178.

Chapter 5 (by subtopic)

Vit C Ester

Bissett, D. L., R. Chatterjee, D. P. Hannon. Photoprotective effect of superoxide-scavenging antioxidants against ultraviolet radiation-induced chronic skin damage in the hairless mouse. *Photodermatol Photoimmunol Photomed.* 1990 Apr.; 7(2): 56–62.

Perricone, N., K. Nagy, F. Horvath, G. Dajko, I. Uray, I. Zs-Nagy. The hydroxyl free radical reactions of ascorbyl palmitate as measured in various in vitro models. *Biochem Biophys Res Commun.* 1999, Sep. 7; 262(3): 661–665.

Perricone, N. V. Photoprotective and anti-inflammatory effects of topical ascorbyl palmitate. *J Geriatr Dermatol.* 1993; 1(1): 5–10.

———. Topical vitamin C ester (ascorbyl palmitate). *J Geriatr Dermatol* 1997; 5(4): 162–170.

———. Topical vitamin C ester (ascorbyl palmitate). Adapted from the first annual symposium on aging skin, San Diego, CA, February 21–23, 1997. *J Geriatric Dermatol.* 1997; 5(4): 162–170.

———. Treatment of psoriasis with topical ascorbyl palmitate. *Clinical Research.* 1991; 39: 535A.

Rosenblat, G., et al. Acylated ascorbate stimulates collagen synthesis in cultured human foreskin fibroblasts at lower doses than does ascorbic acid. *Connect Tissue Res.* 1998; 37(3–4): 303–311.

Smart, R. C., and C. L. Crawford. Effect of ascorbic acid and its synthetic lipophilic derivative ascorbyl palmitate on phorbol ester-induced skin-tumor promotion in mice. *Am J Clin Nutr.* 1991 Dec.; 54(6 Suppl): 1266S–1273S.

Tebbe, B., S. Wu, C. C. Geilen, J. Eberle, V. Kodelja, and C. E. Orfanos. L-ascorbic acid inhibits UVA-induced lipid peroxidation and secretion of IL-1alpha and IL-6 in cultured human keratinocytes in vitro. *J Invest Dermatol.* 1997 Mar.; 108(3): 302–306.

ALA

Bierhaus, A., et al. Advanced glycation end product-induced activation of NF-kappaB is suppressed by alpha-lipoic acid in cultured endothelial cells. *Diabetes.* 1997 Sep.; 46(9): 1481–1490.

Fuchs, J., and R. Milbradt. Antioxidant inhibition of skin inflammation induced by reactive oxidants: Evaluation of the redox couple dihydrolipoate/lipoate. *Skin Pharmacol.* 1994; 7(5): 278–284.

Fuchs, J., L. Packer, and G. Zimmer. *Lipoic Acid in Health and Disease.* New York: Marcel Dekker, 1997.

Genecov, D. G., K. E. Salyer, M. A. Kemer, S. Goldberg, and J. Cho. Alpha lipoic acid (ALA) and scar formation in repaired cleft lips. International Society of Cleft Lip and Palate. 2001 June; 462: 495–499.

Kagan, V. E., A. Shvedova, E. Serbinova, S. Khan, C. Swanson, R. Powell, and L. Packer. Dihydrolipoic acid—A universal antioxidant both in the membrane and in the aqueous phase. Reduction of peroxyl, ascorbyl and chromanoxyl radicals. *Biochem Pharmacol.* 1992, Oct. 20; 44(8): 1637–1649.

Kunt, T., et al. Alpha-lipoic acid reduces expression of vascular cell adhesion molecule-1 and endothelial adhesion of human monocytes after stimulation with advanced glycation end products. *Clin Sci* (London). 1999 Jan.; 96(1): 75–82.

Meyer, M., H. L. Pahl, and P. A. Baeuerle. Regulation of the transcription factors NF-kappa B and AP-1 by redox changes. *Chem Biol Interact.* 1994 Jun.; 91(2–3): 91–100.

Meyer, M., R. Schreck, and P. A. Baeuerle. H_2O_2 and antioxidants have opposite effects on activation of NF-kappa B and AP-1 in intact cells: AP-1 as secondary antioxidant-responsive factor. *EMBO J.* 1993 May; 12(5): 2005–2015.

Packer, L., S. Roy, and C. K. Sen. A-Lipoic acid: A metabolic antioxidant and potential redox modulator of transcription. *Advances in Pharmacology.* 1996; 38: 79–101.

Saliou, C., M. Kitazawa, L. McLaughlin, J. P. Yang, J. K. Lodge, T. Tetsuka, K. Iwasaki, J. Cillard, T. Okamoto, and L. Packer. Antioxidants modulate acute solar ultraviolet radiation-induced NF-kappa-B activation in a human keratinocyte cell line. *Free Radic Biol Med.* 1999 Jan.; 26(1–2): 174–183.

Sen, C. K., and L. Packer. Antioxidant and redox regulation of gene transcription. *FASEB J.* 1996; 10: 709–720.

Suzuki, Y. J., B. B. Aggarwal, and L. Packer. Alpha-lipoic acid is a potent inhibitor of NF-kappa B activation in human T cells. *Biochem Biophys Res Commun.* 1992, Dec. 30; 189(3): 1709–1715.

Suzuki, Y. J., M. Mizuno, H. J. Tritschler, and L. Packer. Redox regulation of NF-kappa B DNA binding activity by dihydrolipoate. *Biochem Mol Biol Int.* 1995 Jun.; 36(2): 241–246.

DMAE

Alkadhi, K. A. Endplate channel actions of a hemicholinium-3 analog, DMAE. *Naunyn Schmiedebergs Arch Pharmacol.* 1986 Mar.; 332(3): 230–235.

Alvaro, D., A. Cantafora, C. Gandin, R. Masella, M. T. Santini, and M. Angelico. Selective hepatic enrichment of polyunsaturated phosphatidylcholines after intravenous administration of dimethylethanolamine in the rat. *Biochim Biophys Acta.* 1989, Nov. 6; 1006(1): 116–120.

Cole, A. C., E. M. Gisoldi, and R. M. Grossman. Clinical and consumer evaluations of improved facial appearance after 1 month use of topical dimethylaminoethanol. Poster presentation, American Academy of Dermatology, 2002, Feb. 22–26, New Orleans, USA.

Grossman, R. M., E. M. Gisoldi, and A. C. Cole. Long-term safety and efficacy evaluation of a new skin firming technology: Dimethylaminoethanol. Poster presentation, American Academy of Dermatology, 2002, Feb. 22–26, New Orleans, USA.

Guyton, A. C. "Contraction of Skeletal Muscle," ch. 11 in *Textbook of Medical Physiology;* pp. 131–147. Philadelphia: W. B. Saunders Co., 1971.

Nagy, I., and R. A. Floyd. Electron spin resonance spectroscopic demonstration of the hydroxyl free radical scavenger properties of dimethylaminoethanol in spin trapping experiments confirming the molecular basis for the biological effects of centrophenoxine. *Arch Gerontol Geriatr.* 1984 Dec.; 3(4): 297–310.

Nagy, I., and K. Nagy. On the role of cross-linking of cellular proteins in aging. *Mech Ageing Dev.* 1980 Sep.–Oct.; 14(1–2): 245–251.

Perricone, N. V. Topical vitamin C ester (ascorbyl palmitate). Adapted from the first annual symposium on aging skin, San Diego, CA, February 21–23, 1997. *J Geriatric Dermatol.* 1997; 5(4): 162–170.

Semsei, I., and I. Zs-Nagy. Superoxide radical scavenging ability of centrophenoxine and its salt dependence in vitro. *J Free Radic Biol Med.* 1985; 1(5–6): 403–408.

Stryer, L. *Biochemistry, 3rd Edition.* San Francisco: W. H. Freeman and Co., 1988.

Yu, M. J., et al. Phenothiazines as lipid peroxidation inhibitors and cytoprotective agents. *J Med Chem.* 1992, Feb. 21; 35(4): 716–724.

Zs-Nagy, I. On the role of intracellular physicochemistry in quantitative gene expression during aging and the effect of centrophenoxine. A review. *Arch Gerontol Geriatr.* 1989 Nov.–Dec.; 9(3): 215–229.

Zs-Nagy, I., and I. Semsei. Centrophenoxine increases the rates of total and mRNA synthesis in the brain cortex of old rats: An explanation of its action in terms of the membrane hypothesis of aging. *Exp Gerontol.* 1984; 19(3): 171–178.

PPC

Aleynik, S. I., M. A. Leo, M. K. Aleynik, and C. S. Lieber. Alcohol-induced pancreatic oxidative stress: Protection by phospholipid repletion. *Free Radic Biol Med.* 1999 Mar.; 26(5–6): 609–619.

————. Polyenylphosphatidylcholine opposes the increase of cytochrome P-4502E1 by ethanol and corrects its iron-induced decrease. *Alcohol Clin Exp Res.* 1999 Jan.; 23(1): 96–100.

————. Polyenylphosphatidylcholine protects against alcohol but not iron-induced oxidative stress in the liver. *Alcohol Clin Exp Res.* 2000 Feb.; 24(2): 196–206.

Aleynik, S. I., M. A. Leo, U. Takeshige, M. K. Aleynik, and C. S. Lieber. Dilinoleoylphosphatidylcholine is the active antioxidant of polyenylphosphatidylcholine. *J Investig Med.* 1999 Nov.; 47(9): 507–512.

Lichtenberger, L. M., J. J. Romero, W. M. de Ruijter, F. Behbod, R. Darling, A. O. Ashraf, and S. K. Sanduja. Phosphatidylcholine association increases the anti-inflammatory and analgesic activity of ibuprofen in acute and chronic rodent models of joint inflammation: Relationship to alterations in bioavailability and cyclooxygenase-inhibitory potency. *J Pharmacol Exp Ther.* 2001 Jul.; 298(1): 279–287.

TOCOTRIENOLS

Serbinova, E., V. Kagan, D. Han, and L. Packer. Free radical recycling and intramembrane mobility in the antioxidant properties of alpha-tocopherol and alpha-tocotrienol. *Free Radic Biol Med.* 1991; 10(5): 263–275.

Serbinova, E. A., and L. Packer. Antioxidant properties of alpha-tocopherol and alpha-tocotrienol. *Methods Enzymol.* 1994; 234: 354–366.

Thiele, J. J., M. G. Traber, and L. Packer. Depletion of human stratum corneum vitamin E: An early and sensitive in vivo marker of UV induced photooxidation. *J Invest Dermatol.* 1998 May; 110(5): 756–761.

Traber, M. G., M. Rallis, M. Podda, C. Weber, H. I. Maibach, and L. Packer. Penetration and distribution of alpha-tocopherol, alpha- or gamma-tocotrienols applied individually onto murine skin. *Lipids.* 1998 Jan.; 33(1): 87–91.

Traber, M. G., et al. Diet derived topically applied tocotrienols accumulate in skin and protect the tissue against UV light-induced oxidative stress. *Asia Pacific Journal of Clinical Nutrition.* 1997; 6: 63–67.

OOP

Briante, R., F. La Cara, M. P. Tonziello, F. Febbraio, and R. Nucci. Antioxidant activity of the main bioactive derivatives from oleuropein hydrolysis by hyperthermophilic beta-glycosidase. *J Agric Food Chem.* 2001 Jul.; 49(7): 3198–3203.

D'Angelo, S., C. Manna, V. Migliardi, O. Mazzoni, P. Morrica, G. Capasso, G. Pontoni, P. Galletti, and V. Zappia. Pharmacokinetics and metabolism of hydroxytyrosol, a natural antioxidant from olive oil. *Drug Metab Dispos.* 2001 Nov.; 29(11): 1492–1498.

de la Puerta, R., M. F. Martinez Dominguez, V. Ruiz-Gutierrez, J. A. Flavill, and J. R. Hoult. Effects of virgin olive oil phenolics on scavenging of reactive nitrogen species and upon nitrergic neurotransmission. *Life Sci.* 2001, Jul. 27; 69(10): 1213–1222.

Gordon, M. H., F. Paiva-Martins, and M. Almeida. Antioxidant activity of hydroxytyrosol acetate compared with that of other olive oil polyphenols. *J Agric Food Chem.* 2001 May; 49: (5) 2480–2485.

Tuck, K. L., M. P. Freeman, P. J. Hayball, G. L. Stretch, and I. Stupans. The in vivo fate of hydroxytyrosol and tyrosol, antioxidant phenolic constituents of olive oil, after intravenous and oral dosing of labeled compounds to rats. *J Nutr.* 2001 Jul.; 131(7): 1993–1996.

Visioli, F., A. Poli, and C. Gall. Antioxidant and other biological activities of phenols from olives and olive oil. *Med Res Rev.* 2002 Jan.; 22(1): 65–75.

Chapter 6

Fielding, R. A., and M. Meydani. Exercise, free radical generation, and aging. *Aging* (Milano). 1997 Feb.–Apr.; 9(1–2): 12–18.

Haennel, R. G., and F. Lemire Physical activity to prevent cardiovascular disease. How much is enough? *Can Fam Physician.* 2002 Jan.; 48: 65–71.

Ji, L. L. Exercise at old age: Does it increase or alleviate oxidative stress? *Ann NY Acad Sci.* 2001 Apr.; 928: 236–247.

Kasch, F. W., J. L. Boyer, S. P. Van Camp, L. S. Verity, and J. P. Wallace. Effect of exercise on cardiovascular ageing. *Age Ageing.* 1993 Jan.; 22(1): 5–10.

Pansarasa, O., L. Castagna, B. Colombi, J. Vecchiet, G. Felzani, and F. Marzatico. Age and sex differences in human skeletal muscle: Role of reactive oxygen species. *Free Radic Res.* 2000 Sep.; 33(3): 287–293.

Radak, Z., A. W. Taylor, H. Ohno, and S. Goto. Adaptation to exercise-induced oxidative stress: From muscle to brain. *Exerc Immunol Rev.* 2001; 7: 90–107.

Rall, L. C., R. Roubenoff, J. G. Cannon, L. W. Abad, C. A. Dinarello, and S. N. Meydani. Effects of progressive resistance training on immune response in aging and chronic inflammation. *Med Sci Sports Exerc.* 1996 Nov.; 28(11): 1356–1365.

Chapter 7

CORTISOL

Black, M. M., N. E. Platt, and C. J. Mugglestone. A study of potential skin atrophy following topical application of weak corticosteroids. *Curr Med Res Opin.* 1981; 7(7): 463–470.

Cao, G., R. M. Russell, N. Lischner, and R. L. Prior. Serum antioxidant capacity is increased by consumption of strawberries, spinach, red wine or vitamin C in elderly women. *J Nutr.* 1998.

Cole, A. C., E. M. Gisoldi, and R. M. Grossman. Clinical and consumer evaluations of improved facial appearance after 1 month use of topical dimethylaminoethanol. Poster presentation, American Academy of Dermatology, 2002, Feb. 22–26; New Orleans, USA.

Crowley, M. A., and K. S. Matt. Hormonal regulation of skeletal muscle hypertrophy in rats: The testosterone to cortisol ratio. *Eur J Appl Physiol Occup Physiol.* 1996; 73(1–2): 66–72.

Ferrari, E., D. Casarotti, B. Muzzoni, N. Albertelli, L. Cravello, M. Fioravanti, S. B. Solerte and F. Magri. Age-related changes of the adrenal secretory pattern: Possible role in pathological brain aging. *Brain Res Rev.* 2001 Nov.; 37(1–3): 294–300.

Grossman, R. M., E. M. Gisoldi, and A. C. Cole. Long-term safety and efficacy evaluation of a new skin firming technology: Dimethylaminoethanol. Poster presentation, American Academy of Dermatology. 2002, Feb. 22–26; New Orleans, USA.

Heffelfinger, A. K., and J. W. Newcomer. Glucocorticoid effects on memory function over the human life span. *Dev Psychopathol.* 2001 Summer; 13(3): 491–513.

Mazzoccoli, G., M. Correra, G. Bianco, A. De Cata, M. Balzanelli, A. Giuliani, and R. Tarquini. Age-related changes of neuro-endocrine-immune interactions in healthy humans. *J Biol Regul Homeost Agents.* 1997 Oct.–Dec.; 11(4): 143–147.

Stone, B. M. and C. Turner. Promoting sleep in shiftworkers and intercontinental travelers. *Chronobiol Int.* 1997 Mar.; 14(2): 133–143.

Tammi, R. A histometric and autoradiographic study of hydrocortisone action in cultured human epidermis. *Br J Dermatol.* 1981 Oct.; 105(4): 383–389.

Uno, H., S. Eisele, A. Sakai, S. Shelton, E. Baker, O. DeJesus, and J. Holden. Neurotoxicity of glucocorticoids in the primate brain. *Horm Behav.* 1994 Dec.; 28(4): 336–348.

U.S. Department of Agriculture, Agricultural Research Service. USDA Nutrient Database for Standard Reference, Release 14. 2001. Nutrient Data Laboratory Home Page: http://www.nal.usda.gov/fnic/foodcomp

Wang, S. Y., and H. S. Lin. Antioxidant activity in fruits and leaves of blackberry, raspberry, and strawberry varies with cultivar and developmental stage. *J Agric Food Chem.* 2000 Feb.; 48(2): 140–146.

Zheng, W., and S. Y. Wang. Antioxidant activity and phenolic compounds in selected herbs. *J Agric Food Chem.* 2001 Nov.; 49(11): 5165–5170.

Chapter 8

Althaus, J. S., T. J. Fleck, D. A. Becker, E. D. Hall, and P. F. Vonvoigtlander. Azulenyl nitrones: Colorimetric detection of oxyradical end products and neuroprotection in the gerbil transient forebrain ischemia/reperfusion model. *Free Radic Biol Med.* 1998, Mar. 15; 24(5): 738–744.

Becker, D. A. Diagnostic and therapeutic applications of azulenyl nitrone spin traps. *Cell Mol Life Sci.* 1999, Nov. 15; 56(7–8): 626–633.

Bodnar, A. G., M. Ouellette, M. Frolkis, S. E. Holt, C. P. Chiu, G. B. Morin, C. B. Harley, J. W. Shay, S. Lichtsteiner, and W. E. Wright. Extension of lifespan by introduction of telomerase into normal human cells. *Science.* 1998, Jan. 16; 279(5349): 349–352.

Cole, A. C., E. M. Gisoldi, and R. M. Grossman. Clinical and consumer evaluations of improved facial appearance after 1 month use of topical dimethylaminoethanol. Poster presentation, American Academy of Dermatology, 2002, Feb. 22–26; New Orleans, USA.

Ferber, D. Immortalized cells seem cancer-free so far. *Science.* 1999, Jan. 8; 283(5399): 154–155.

Grossman, R. M., E. M. Gisoldi, and A. C. Cole. Long-term safety and efficacy evaluation of a new skin firming technology: Dimethylaminoethanol. Poster presentation, American Academy of Dermatology, 2002, Feb. 22–26; New Orleans, USA.

Klivenyi, P., R. T. Matthews, M. Wermer, L. Yang, U. MacGarvey, D. A. Becker, R. Natero, and M. F. Beal. Azulenyl nitrone spin traps protect against MPTP neurotoxicity. *Exp Neurol.* 1998 Jul.; 152(1): 163–166.

Mak, I. T., A. Murphy, A. Hopper, D. Witiak, J. Ziemniak, and W. B. Weglicki. Potent inhibitory activities of hydrophobic aci-reductones (2-hydroxytetronic acid analogs) against membrane and human low-density lipoprotein oxidation. *Biochem Pharmacol.* 1998, Jun. 1; 55(11): 1921–1926.

Malinda, K. M., G. S. Sidhu, H. Mani, K. Banaudha, R. K. Maheshwari, A. L. Goldstein, and H. K. Kleinman. Thymosin beta4 accelerates wound healing. *J Invest Dermatol.* 1999 Sep.; 113(3): 364–368.

Perez-Bernal, A., M. A. Munoz-Perez, and F. Camacho. Management of facial hyperpigmentation. *Am J Clin Dermatol.* 2000 Sep.–Oct.; 1(5): 261–268.

Sosne, G., C. C. Chan, K. Thai, M. Kennedy, E. A. Szliter, L. D. Hazlett, and H. K. Kleinman. Thymosin beta 4 promotes corneal wound healing and modulates inflammatory mediators in vivo. *Exp Eye Res.* 2001 May; 72(5): 605–608.

Tung, R. C., W. F. Bergfeld, A. T. Vidimos, and B. K. Remzi. Alpha-hydroxy acid-based cosmetic procedures. Guidelines for patient management. *Am J Clin Dermatol.* 2000 Mar.–Apr.; 1(2): 81–88.

Index